What to Do When Antibiotics Don't Work!

How to stay healthy and alive when infections strike

Dirk van Gils

What To Do When Antibiotics Don't Work!

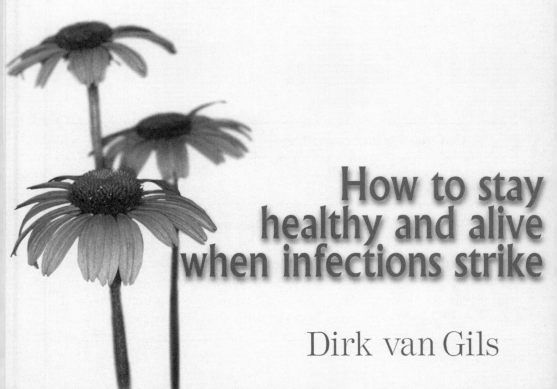

How to stay healthy and alive when infections strike

Dirk van Gils

Library of Congress Control Number: 2002106469

Printed in the United States of America

International Standard Book Number (ISBN)

Paper: 0-9720194-0-5

Published by Health Practice Books
P.O. Box 322
Payson, UT 84651

Acknowledgements

Many people helped make this project a reality.

I am especially grateful to:

My wife Toni, for your genius, vision, and love.

Our children Christine, Sean, Jon Alex, Jennifer, and Gerard, for your examples.

My mother and father, for the journey that brought us here.

Annemarier Buhler, mentor and friend, the first woman to bring essential oil scientific research into the United States. Many will be eternally grateful to you.

Joyce and Scott Beach, Annette Davis, and Cecilia Salvesen for contributing their expertise to this project.

Rachel Gibson and Dale Lott for the cover design, formatting, and editorial assistance in preparing this manuscript.

And to friends and colleagues who answered questions and reviewed the manuscript—Gerard van Gils, Reagan Cox, Dean Dobmeier, Annelle Norman, Dr. Alvin B. Segelman, Ph.D., and Dr. Luba Vozarova, Ph.D.

Preface

The warm South Carolina sky was a robin-egg blue, the air was kissed with the bloom of spring lilacs, and my mother was excited. At the age of 80, she was preparing to embark on her first cruise with a friend.

Over the previous week, though, Mother had become slightly concerned about a recurring, twinge-type of pain in her arm. Her physician of many years could find no reason to worry, but decided that Mother should go for a heart stress test before leaving on her vacation.

Ever the willing candidate to visit a doctor, Mother walked into the office and stepped onto the treadmill at 2:30 p.m. A short time later, she was wheeled out of the same office on a gurney, her last breath unexpectedly spent. She had passed away suddenly from age and causes unknown.

Although not diagnosed as the cause of death, an autopsy revealed the presence of 15 different prescription medications present in Mother's tissues and organs. The physician performing the autopsy was surprised with this finding, but I was not.

Like so many others raised in a time when people thought science and medicine could do no wrong, I grew up in a home where doctor's appointments and prescription medications were constant companions, even friends. My mother used antibiotics for yeast infections, earaches, and the common scratchy throat. When one antibiotic stopped working for her, she would try another. Somehow, she always seemed to have a supply of antibiotics on hand. Mother used muscle relaxants for migraine headaches, Valium when she was depressed, and various pain pills for everything else.

My mother was a determined person. Her belief system in antibiotics and other medications was strong. I cannot remember a time when she did not rely completely on prescription medications to "keep her going." She never considered alternative methods of healing—perhaps she did not even know there were options.

"But," you might be thinking, "your mother *did* live to be 80 years of age."

That's true, but her quality of life was never what it might have been. All the years of stressing her body and depressing her immune system with prescriptions took a physical, emotional, and financial toll on her and all of us who knew her. Mother was continually troubled with yeast infections, earaches, migraines, depression, eye irritation, and various bacterial and viral infections. Over the years she came to believe that it was her "lot in life" to be sick. It need not have been that way.

My point in telling this is a simple one—take the opportunity to learn before it is too late. Don't suppress the warning signals your body gives you by smothering them with medications. Address the root causes of your illness. Your body wants to be healthy, and you have a divine right to a healthy life.

What To Do When Antibiotics Don't Work may well become one of the most important books in your library. I know you will reference it over and over. When you do, please remember the people in your circle who could use an alternative to the same old regime of expensive medications that never quite seem to do the trick.

I know the information in this book will bless your life.

Toni van Gils

June, 2002

Contents

Acknowledgements 5

Preface 7

Contents 9

Introduction 11

Chapter 1—What Are Plant Medicines? 15

Chapter 2—Natural Antibiotics 29

Chapter 3—Why Use Plant Medicines? 44

Chapter 4—Understanding Infections 56

Chapter 5—How To Use Plant Medicines 73

Chapter 6—When Infections Strike 88

    Abscesses 90

    Acne 91

    Anthrax 93

    Athlete's Foot, Nail Fungus, Ringworm 95

    Bites and Stings 97

    Boils 101

    Bronchitis 102

    Bubonic Plague 106

    Candida Albicans 108

    Chicken Pox 110

    Colitis 111

    Common Cold 115

    Cystitis 117

    Diarrhea 120

    Ear Infections 121

    Eczema 123

    Eye Infections 125

    Fevers 127

    Gall Bladder Inflammation 130

    Gastritis 132

    Headaches 133

    Hepatitis 135

    Herpes Simplex 137

    HIV Support 140

    Impetigo 142

Influenza 143
Intestinal Parasites and Worms 145
Kidney Infection 148
Lice Infestation 149
Lyme Disease 150
Measles 152
Mouth Infections 155
Mumps 157
Muscle Aches and Pains 159
Pneumonia 160
Prostatitis 161
Psoriasis 162
Scarlet Fever 163
Shingles 165
Sinusitis 167
Sore Throat 169
Testicular Infection 170
Tonsillitis 171
Tuberculosis 173
Urethritis 174
Vaginitis 176
Warts 178
Whooping Cough 179
Wound Healing 181
Glossary 185
Appendix A—Essential Oil List 187
Appendix B—Herb List 191
Notes 197

Introduction

"...The misuse of antibiotics leads to numerous side effects and sometimes results in chronic disastrous conditions...that could have been avoided if medical aromatherapy had been implemented." —Shirley Price

Welcome to *What To Do When Antibiotics Don't Work!* The purpose of this book is to provide you with clear, concise directions on what to do to preserve your health and your life when antibiotic drugs are ineffective, inappropriate, or unavailable. Because of world conditions and the growth of antibiotic resistant germs, all of us face the threat of ravaging, epidemic diseases that cause misery and death. There are also situations when antibiotics cannot be used due to a pre-existing condition—such as an allergy or a pregnancy—or when drugs are not available because know-how, resources, or supplies are lacking.

This information is for everyone—not just for those who want to know what to do in case of an epidemic. Many of us suffer on a daily basis with all kinds of illness. Acute, chronic, and recurring infections are among the most frequent problems we face. I will discuss ways to control these problems by boosting your immune system and by treating common infections with essential oils and herbs.

Natural plant medicines have been used throughout human history. They deserve serious study, for their potential as a healing therapy is enormous. Unfortunately, the public today is still largely unfamiliar with how to use plant medicines against infectious diseases. This also holds true for many health care practitioners. In the meantime, the threat from infectious diseases is an ever-growing problem.

How this book came about

I am an author specializing in alternative health care. Last year I completed another writing assignment—a 360-page training manual entitled *Aromatherapy and the Whole Body*—to assist my wife, who is an aromatherapy educator for a large, international company.

At some point during the course of that project, we were talking about French doctors and how they use herbal medicines to fight infections. "In France today," wrote Julia Lawless, an expert in aromatherapy, "many medical doctors and hospitals prescribe essential oils as an alternative to antibiotic treatment, whereas in most other countries the idea of using natural aromatics as a form of medical treatment is still very radical."[1] This concept intrigued me, so I ordered several medical aromatherapy books from France. (My years of studying French were paying off!)

What I read excited me. In France, many trained medical doctors use essential oils and herbs to fight common infections. They are primarily used for respiratory infections, but they are also useful against infections of the digestive system, the urinary tract, the reproductive organs, and the skin. Essential oils and herbs can be used as the primary treatment method, or—depending on patient characteristics and the nature of the illness—they can be used in conjunction with antibiotics and other treatment modalities. French doctors do not limit themselves to practicing only herbal medicine, but incorporate the full extent of modern medical knowledge and skill into their approach to medical care.

The French are world leaders in the field of aromatherapy, the use of essential oils for therapeutic purposes. Since medical aromatherapy treatments are considered normal and routine, treatments using herbs and essential oils are covered by health insurance plans. People in France can go to pharmacies where formulas consisting of essential oils and herbal tinctures are specifically made under a doctor's prescription. Medical aromatherapy is taught in colleges, universities, and medical schools. There are also important regional and national aromatherapy associations, and the French are taking the lead in disseminating aromatherapy research worldwide.

Herbal medicine in the United States

In the United States, natural plant medicines are commonly available, but medical doctors rarely use them to treat infections. The American public in general is unfamiliar with aromatherapy. Most people have never even smelled an essential oil, and if they did, they would not be able to tell the difference between a genuine essential oil and a commercial "fragrance"—much less how they should be used. In the U.S., aromatherapy is associated with the "new age" movement or the products found in shops that sell candles, scents, and bath and body care products. The possibility of using essential oils for medicinal purposes is not well understood.

This happens in part because plant medicines are not given the same regulatory stature as conventional prescription drugs. Instead, plant medicines are often called "alternative" or "natural" medicines. The terms "integrative" or "complementary" medicine are also sometimes linked to plant medicine. Although natural medicine is growing in popularity and acceptance, official recognition and support are still lacking.

For this reason, herbal medicines are not regarded seriously enough by the public or by the medical and political establishment. U.S. medical students do not receive training in how to use essential oils and herbs in treating infections. Instead, the treatment focus of conventional medicine is not on health care, but on treating illnesses and symptoms with prescription drugs and invasive procedures that involve surgery. There is little emphasis on preventive care or nutrition. Few insurance programs that will cover the costs of alternative health care are available to patients. There is comparatively little public or private funding available for natural health care research. Even training and licensing requirements for alternative health care practitioners can vary widely from state to state.

Natural plant medicines

Natural plant medicines are safe, comparatively inexpensive, practical to use, quick acting, and effective against infections. The use of plant medicines to combat infections is adequately documented in the medical and scientific literature. There is now also ample clinical experience to show how plant medicines can be effective for a wide range of health problems caused by infections.

Unfortunately, much of the relevant research is not readily available in the U.S. Most of the research and medical literature available on this topic is available only in other countries. I have drawn on that literature to prepare this book. The methods of treatment presented here model those of the French, who emphasize the combined use of essential oils and herbal tinctures in treating infections.

As far as I am aware, this is the first time a book totally dedicated to fighting infections by combining the use of essential oils with herbs has been written in English.

Why I wrote this book

This book was written in the belief that good health is a professional and personal responsibility.

I do not advocate self-care in the treatment of infectious diseases. Some advocates of natural medicine tend to shy away from doctors, but this is a mistake. Serious ailments, including many infectious illnesses, should be reported to a skillful health care professional and treated under his or her supervision. There are valid reasons for doing so, and they are explained in this book.

However, each of us is ultimately responsible for our own health and well-being and the choices we make. In order to make better decisions, people should be informed about alternative treatments and what they can do to live a longer and healthier life. A freely informed public is in everyone's best interest.

This book also has been written with the hope that it will help people stay healthy and alive. Because many are sick and dying needlessly, my goal is to make people aware that there is a viable alternative when conventional treatments do not work. If the information found here is used only once to save a life, then your investment in reading this book will have been priceless.

Welcome to the exciting world of herbal medicine!

Chapter 1
What Are Plant Medicines?

"Any person who ventures into the world of aromatherapy should be given a symbolic key, as this experience opens a door to a new world—a world we did not realize existed. Lemon is no longer seen as a garnish, but a strong antiseptic which treats infection. Garlic is no longer a herb which flavors food, but the realization that it's nature's antibiotic quickly sets in. Black pepper is not merely a delight for steak lovers, but a powerful circulatory stimulant, and clove an analgesic rather than a decoration on an orange."
—Cecilia Salvesen

Simply stated, *plant medicines* are medicines made from plants. The terms *phytotherapy* (plant therapy) or *herbal medicine* may also be used. Plant medicines are obtained from many types of plants, not just herbs.

Aromatherapy, the therapeutic use of essential oils, is a branch of plant medicine. Essential oils were used anciently, but their medicinal use was largely overlooked or forgotten until French physicians rediscovered them in the past century.

Plant medicines are obtained from many varieties of plants, flowers, grasses, herbs, fruits, and trees. They have a long history of being recognized for their therapeutic qualities. Plants have been used in the healing arts for thousands of years.

Prehistoric graves have been uncovered by archaeologists that contain medical plants buried alongside human skeletal remains. The Chinese have been cultivating useful medicinal plants for at least 4,500 years. Vedic literature originating in present-day India dates from 2000 B.C. and lists more than 700 plant materials for medicinal use, including Cinnamon, Spikenard, Ginger, Myrrh, Coriander, and Sandalwood. Medicinal plants are mentioned in the Bible and the Koran. Plant medicine forms part of every cultural tradition.

The first Americans to use herbal medicines were the American Indians. When the Spanish and Portuguese colonized South America, they discovered some of the world's most important medicinal plants—Cinchona Bark and Ipecacuanha. Quinine, an anti-malarial drug, was derived from Cinchona Bark. Ipecac, a drug used to induce vomiting, was obtained from the dried root of the Ipecacuanha plant growing in Brazil.

As early as 1534, Indians living in Canada along the St. Lawrence seaway showed the French how to counteract scurvy by boiling a mixture of pine needles and bark from the white pine tree, a plant rich in Vitamin C. But the French did not listen to the Indians; they believed that the natives were ignorant savages. European sailors continued dying from scurvy until well into the nineteenth century.

During colonial times, American Indians taught pioneers how to use Native American herbs and plants. American Indians preferred using the roots and bark of plants, rather than the flowers, leaves, seeds, and aerial parts as was the custom in Europe.[1] Colonial physicians used American Indian plants to cure camp fevers during the revolutionary war because European preparations were then unavailable.[2] By the same token, white settlers brought their own herbal traditions to America and eventually taught these to the Indians.

The herbal medicines we use in America today originate with our diverse American Indian and immigrant heritage. Examples of Indian medicinal herbs include Black Cohosh, used by the Eastern Woodland Indians and later by colonial settlers for menstrual disorders; Black Walnut, used for constipation, impacted bowels, and to expel parasites and worms; and Goldenrod, which was for colds, fever, flu, and respiratory conditions.[3] Medicinal plants found natively in America include Echinacea, Garlic, Goldenseal, Ginseng, Ginkgo Biloba, Saw Palmetto, Aloe Vera, Bayberry, Bearberry, Bilberry, Cascara Sagrada, Cranberry, Slippery Elm, St. John's Wort, and White Oak. Most of these herbs are suitable in the treatment of infections and are still in use today.

Echinacea is now probably the most widely sold herbal medicine in the United States. It was originally used by the North American Plains Indians, who used the root of the plant as a snake bite remedy. In the 1880s, a patent remedy vendor in Nebraska, Dr. H.C.F. Meyer, learned about Echinacea from Indians and began promoting it as a cure-all. He claimed to have cured hundreds of snake bites with Echinacea and at times allowed himself to be bitten by a snake in order to demonstrate the plant's healing powers. This was the original "snake oil remedy."[4]

During the years that followed, Echinacea came to be used by doctors as a treatment for septicemia (blood infection). They used it as a cure for abscesses, boils, carbuncles, tissue inflammation, gangrene, and many other related illnesses.

When pharmaceutical drugs became popular in the twentieth century, the use of herbal medicines declined in the United States. A limited number of homeopaths and natural care practitioners continued prescribing Echinacea, but the public's familiarity with the plant was lost.[5]

Following World War II, a pharmaceutical firm in Germany obtained Echinacea from America and began investigating the plant's medicinal properties. The Germans published several research studies. In one of them, 203 women with recurring vaginal yeast infections were treated with either a standard pharmaceutical cream or the cream plus oral doses of Echinacea. The group treated only with cream suffered 60% recurring infections within six months. Among those who also took Echinacea, that figure was only 16%—a considerable difference in results.[6]

During the "herbal revival" of the 1970s, Echinacea became popular in Germany, and soon after was reintroduced to the North American market. Countless other studies were conducted demonstrating the plant's impressive healing properties. Today the medicinal effects of Echinacea are well known. It is commonplace to find doctors recommending it for use during a cold, the flu, or for other types of illnesses. A similar story may be told about other plant medicines once people understand their value.

What are essential oils?

Essential oils are the by-product or end result of *plant metabolism,* the biological activity of plants. They are synthesized by the plant's chemistry and circulate through the stems, leaves, flowers, and roots. They contain the elements that make each plant unique — the scent and the intelligence of the plant. Walk through a forest of pine trees and you can easily smell their fragrance. Essential oils are found in the skin of an orange, in the leaves of a peppermint plant, and in the petals of a rose flower. Essential oils give the plant its aroma and flavor. When they are properly used as medicines they can have a significant physiological effect on the body.

Essential oils are "essential" for a plant's survival. Scientists have observed that different varieties of plants use essential oils to repel unwanted insects, to help in healing the plant when the plant has been injured, to prevent water loss from foliage when the climate is hot or dry, or to attract bees and other insects that aid in pollination. Essential oils are a key component of the immune system of plants.[7]

Essential oils are stored by plants in oil and resin ducts, hollow spaces and cells. They can be found in the leaves and stems of plants, flowers, fruits; and in the skin of fruits, herbs, grasses, and trees (in wood, twigs, bark, needles, and resins).

With few exceptions, essential oils are extracted from plant materials through *cold pressing* or *distillation*. Cold pressing is used to remove citrus oils from the peel of citrus fruits such as grapefruit, orange, lemon, lime, and tangerine. Distillation is used to produce most other oils.

Distillation is accomplished by using water or steam, but there are different types of distillation methods. The oldest method of distillation is to place plant material in a still, cover the plant material with water, and bring it to a certain temperature. The essential oils then separate from the plant. They do not mix with water because they are only fat-soluble.

When an essential oil is distilled, each plant has unique requirements in terms of how the plant should be handled. These include when to harvest, time between harvesting and distillation, distillation equipment, temperature, pressure, and when to stop distillation in order to avoid exposing the essential oil to excessive heat, thus destroying vital constituents or medicinal properties.

Thousands of tons of essential oils are used each year by the flavor and fragrance industry. This industry uses essential oils in foods and in personal care products such as shampoo, hair conditioner, toothpaste, mouthwash, soap, candles, and perfumes. The essential oils used by this industry are commercial or food grade essential oils. They are inferior in quality to the essential oils used in medical aromatherapy, and cannot be used for therapeutic purposes.

The market for therapeutic essential oils is considerably smaller than the flavor and fragrance market. A small number of independent distillers produce essential oils for use in medical aromatherapy. Because the market for therapeutic essential oils is so small, and because there are relatively few producers, it is not difficult to learn the "genealogy" of essential oils or about where these oils originate. In contrast, commercial oils for the flavor and fragrance industry are sometimes traded four times or more in successive transactions before they are actually used in manufacturing. Agents who transact business in the enormous flavor and fragrance industry are strictly impersonal commodity brokers.

While commercial oils in the flavor and fragrance industry are routinely blended and redistilled for consistency, essential oils used in medical aromatherapy should remain unaltered from their natural state. Therapeutic essential oils—with very few exceptions—should be raw, free from any added substances, unaltered, and genuine. They should also be single-species essential oils, which means that the oil in the bottle contains only the distillation of a single plant species.

Why is this so? Because plants called by a common name can actually represent different plant species. Botanists use botanical names to classify plants into a plant family, a group or *genus*, and then specific species within the genus. For example, Lavender belongs to the *Labiatae* family, the genus *lavandula*, and within *lavandula* there are some 30 different species of Lavender. Each of these have different chemical constituents and medicinal characteristics. On the open market, their quality and price can vary greatly, and certain ones are only used in the flavor and fragrance industry.

For producing medicinal essential oils, the following Lavender species are most commonly used: True Lavender or *Lavandula angustifolia* (syn. *Lavandula vera*), Spike Lavender or *L. latifolia*, Lavandin or *L. hybrida*, and Stoechas Lavender or *L. stoechas*. If the distillations from these different plant species are mixed together and sold under the generic name "Lavender Oil," it becomes difficult to know with certainty what medicinal effect, if any, this mixture will have. In contrast, the therapeutic qualities of a single species such as *Lavandula angustifolia* are predictable because the oil's characteristics are fully documented and well understood.

When purchasing medicinal essential oils, insist on purchasing the species that produces the best medicinal results. There may be a considerable difference in price between True Lavender (*L. angustifolia*) and Lavandin (*L. hybrida*), but this difference is meaningless if the less costly essential oil has few therapeutic properties.

Furthermore, essential oils used for medicinal purposes should be free from all man-made chemicals including contaminants such as herbicides and pesticides. The term "organic" is often used in this context, but the term can mislead as well as inform. "Organic" does not necessarily mean "therapeutic." If a plant has been grown and harvested correctly, has therapeutic properties, and the essential oil from that plant has been distilled correctly, then certified organically grown essential oils are always preferred. But if any of those elements are missing, the plant is of little use even though it is labeled organic.

Organic certification involves regulation and standards set by a governing authority. For example, the state of California has become recognized for its certification standards. Worldwide, many governmental bodies are developing similar standards. An effort is being made to improve standards regulating how organically produced products can be marketed and sold.

This process is still ongoing. Many essential oils are grown in places where there are no procedures in place for designating organically grown plants. Therefore, it is not always possible to designate an essential oil as "organic." Unfortunately, not all manufacturers of herbal products adhere to correct labeling standards. While some companies are very conscientious about correctly labeling their products, others are not. The secret to obtaining essential oils of good quality is to locate a reliable source, a provider who adheres to sound manufacturing and labeling standards.

Physical characteristics of essential oils

Essential oils are highly concentrated plant medicines! It takes more than 100 pounds of eucalyptus leaves to produce 1 pound of eucalyptus essential oil. Two thousand pounds of rose petals produce only 1 liter of essential oil. One drop of peppermint essential oil is the equivalent of approximately 30 cups of peppermint tea!

Essential oils are:
- Liquids
- Lipophilic—they are soluble in fats
- Aromatic—they have an odor
- Volatile—they evaporate easily
- Composed of very small molecules

Most essential oils are not soluble in water, but will dissolve in alcohol. All essential oils are totally soluble in each other. *Carrier oils* are vegetable oils that are able to mix with essential oils. Some texts refer to them as *base oils*. Since most essential oils should not be used undiluted, carrier oils are required along with essential oils in most medical applications. Plants distilled to make carrier oils include common vegetable oils such as Aloe Vera, Jojoba, Grapeseed, Olive, Sweet Almond, or Wheat Germ. (Mineral oils—including baby oil—are derived from petroleum and **are not suitable** for use with essential oils.[8]) Although we refer to them as essential oils, they are not oily to the touch and they leave no greasy residue on the skin.

Chemical characteristics

When chemists study essential oil constituents, they discover that these oils are extremely complex substances. "Chemists have identified more than 3,000 different aromatic molecules, and new ones are continually being discovered."[9] Most essential oils have between 20 to 50 different chemical constituents, some essential oils have as many as 200.[10] Each constituent forms only a small part of the total amount.

Herbal tinctures and other herbal preparations are equally as complex as essential oils. The chemical relationship between the different compounds found in plants is not well understood.

The constituents that are found in plants are the result of "biosynthetic pathways," or a series of chemical reactions that forms the basis of living matter. Their significance is that they are made by nature, and that they form the basis for biological activity and life. Some of these constituents may be synthesized artificially, but such synthetic compounds cannot be made to work biologically in the same way as the compounds made by nature. Perhaps this is why synthetic oils do not smell like natural oils. In synthetic oils, the known constituents of essential oils are mixed together in the proper amounts. They produce a chemical profile almost identical to the natural substance, but their fragrance is different.[11]

Chemists study the different constituents of essential oils in order to determine their effects. The question chemists ask is, what is the effect of the constituent (active ingredient) on the body? In order to answer this question, they first classify essential oils into different categories, depending on the oils' chemical nature and characteristics. Most essential oils are classified as *terpenes* or *terpenoid compounds*. These contain *functional groups* or chemical families including monoterpenes, alcohols, phenols, aldehydes, ketones, esters, and oxides. A smaller number of essential oils are classified as *phenylpropanes*. Phenylpropanes may also be further subdivided into functional groups.[12]

Classifying essential oils into functional groups contributes to our understanding of how essential oils behave when applied to the body. For example, monoterpenes are considered stimulants; ketones are mucolytic (break down mucous); aldehydes are calming; esters are antispasmodic; oxides are expectorants; and so on. It is evident that certain chemicals found in essential oils have predictable effects.

However, this idea can only be taken so far. Because the chemistry of essential oils is complex, and because hundreds of chemicals are involved, it is difficult to establish a direct link between a major ingredient found in an oil and the therapeutic effects found in the complete oil. Knowing the chemical constituents of an essential oil—the active ingredients— gives us a partial understanding, but not complete predictability.[13]

Essential oils are recognized for their antioxidant, antibacterial, antifungal, antiviral, and anti-inflammatory properties. Essential oils are considered effective in the treatment of infections and respiratory conditions, for improving immune response, for balancing the nervous system, and for helping to alleviate psychological and hormonal imbalances. The usage charts found in the Appendix summarize some of these findings.

Although essential oils are chemically complex they can be understood and used. The best way to understand essential oils is to learn as much about each individual oil as you can from the aromatherapy literature, and then begin using them in your daily life.

What are herbal tinctures?

There are many types of natural plant medicines. In addition to essential oils, there are herbal tinctures, herbal teas, decoctions, vinegars, creams, salves, and syrups, to name a few. Many of these may be used to fight infections. Essential oils and herbal tinctures are the most popular plant medicines.

An *herbal tincture* is a liquid solution that contains soluble plant constituents. The liquid is usually alcohol or a combination of alcohol and water. Alcohol is a preservative that protects the plant extract from deterioration.

A conventional tincture is made by first grinding a fresh or dry herb, reducing it in size in order to create a larger surface area of extraction. Depending on the herb, sometimes the whole plant is used and sometimes only certain parts, such as the root, leaves, or flowers, are used. The herbs can be finely milled or they can be processed through a blender, creating pulp. Dry herbs may be reduced to a coarse powder by rubbing through a screen or electric grinder. The extracting solvent, called the *menstruum* is then added.

Maceration is the process of allowing the herbal materials to soak in the menstruum for a period of time. Normally, three weeks is sufficient time for the menstruum to be thoroughly saturated with the plant's medicinal extracts. Maceration typically occurs at room temperature in a dark place.

Before the tincture can be stored away, the macerating extract must be filter pressed in order to separate the liquid portion from solid plant material. The solid plant material (the *marc*) is then discarded.

In commercial tincturing, be aware that not all liquid herbal extracts are created equal. Manufacturing usually involves a variety of techniques, such as heat and stream extraction, cold pressing, steeping and percolating. Unfortunately, many manufacturers—as a result of their extraction methods—manage to destroy important plant constituents or simply discard them, as listed below:

- Many plant materials are oxidized during extraction, destroying the antioxidant portions of the plant. As a result, these tinctures appear a uniform brown or brown-yellow in color; herbs that are not oxidized have natural colors. Examples include: Bilberry— purple in color, Cat's Claw or Una de Gato—a reddish-orange color, and Angelica or Dong Quai—a yellow color.

- Manufacturers use rubber tubing or plastic equipment instead of stainless steel or glass. These materials permit leeching and contamination. Material from the plastic enters into the herbs, and vice versa. When a different herb is processed using the same equipment, active ingredients from the previously processed herb can contaminate the batch.

- At the end of processing, significant amounts of valuable plant material is discarded. Mineral salts and other potentially valuable constituents may be very important in healing.

Another problem revolves around "standardization." When purchasing a tincture, consumers need to be assured that the product contains the active ingredients normally found in the tincture—and that those ingredients are present in therapeutic amounts. Because herbs are a product of nature, natural variations do occur as a result of climate conditions, soil types, and other natural factors. When different batches of herbs are processed, they may vary in how much of a particular constituent can be found.

These naturally occurring variations normally do not affect the therapeutic value of the plant, as long as constituents are present in their proper proportions, a level beneficial to the body. To assure consistency, some manufacturers will mix different batches of the same processed herb together. However, other suppliers identify specific constituents or active ingredients, then guarantee a specific percentage or amount of that component in their product. They do this by artificially adding ingredients to a product.

This practice, which resembles the pharmaceutical approach to medications, overlooks the following:

- Manufacturers might be wrong as to which active ingredient should be standardized to in a given plant.

- Artificially adding constituents to a preparation in order to reach the "standard" upsets the natural ratio of constituents as found in the whole plant, and is adulteration.

- Unscrupulous operators have been known to artificially add ingredients to herbal distillations that, under normal conditions, would be considered of little worth.

• When artificially adding products, manufacturers usually do so at the front end, or at the start, of the manufacturing process. At completion of the process, however, plant materials are discarded, intentionally or unintentionally ensuring that no one knows for sure if the manufacturer's product claims are true without conducting a formal analysis (an *assay*) of the tincture.

The best herbal manufacturers today have not fallen into any of these traps. Their goal, where possible, is to provide the whole plant with the full spectrum of beneficial constituents, in proper balance, to the consumer. "If it's in the plant, it must be in the bottle" is their philosophy.

Nature does nothing in vain

As we've already seen, scientists have an interest in plants in order to find out what the leading constituents are, what the most active ingredients are, and what medicinal effects are produced by these ingredients. Once these are identified, scientists can extract the active ingredients and deliver them in an isolated and concentrated form as a drug.

This practice of isolating ingredients and then administering them to patients in a concentrated form violates one of the basic tenets of traditional herbal medicine. Since the second century, the Greek physician Claudius Galenus (Galen) taught that "nature does nothing in vain," meaning that there is a reason or purpose for the ways plants have developed.

Plants represent thousands of years of evolution and ecological adaptation. Their complex chemistry is an end product essential to life. In their natural form, different constituents within the plant are in proper balance with each other. In isolation, this proper balance no longer exists.

The "nature does nothing in vain" principle leads to the teaching that plant medicines should either be used in their complete or unadulterated form (in their totality) or not used at all. Galen called this the *Law of Totality* or the *Law of All or Nothing*. This law was commonly accepted throughout medieval times, but fell into disregard in the nineteenth and twentieth centuries with the advent of man-made drugs. Today, with the failure of man-made drugs more evident, the Law of All or Nothing is receiving renewed attention and respect within the scientific community.

Many specialists in plant medicine believe that the therapeutic effects of medicinal plants come from the balance and synergy that results when all of these constituents are combined. Some constituents will always predominate in any given plant, but not all of the plant's characteristics can be accounted for by the constituents that predominate. Trace amounts of any constituent may play a very important role.

In numerous studies, scientists have found that whole plants are very important to human health. They have found that a diet rich in whole fruits and vegetables results in a lower incidence of "lifestyle diseases" such as cancer or heart disease.

Scientists are now beginning to suspect that within the chemistry of plants, other phytonutrients not yet identified may contribute to the beneficial health effects of plants. Or, the chemistry of plants in and of itself may be responsible. In a recent article scientists studying the plant constituent lycopene speculated as follows:

> "Although the antioxidant properties of lycopene are thought to be primarily responsible for its beneficial properties, evidence is accumulating to suggest other mechanisms such as intercellular gap junction communication, hormonal and immune system modulation and metabolic pathways may also be involved."[14]

In other words, plant foods containing lycopene may be beneficial to health, but attributing the beneficial effects to lycopene in and of itself may be an oversimplification. Other factors need to be taken into consideration. This suggests that Galen was right—nature does nothing in vain, and plants should be used in their totality or not at all.

Laws regulating plant medicines

Laws that regulate health care in the U.S. are promulgated by state and federal governments. The Food and Drug Administration (FDA) is the federal agency that regulates medicinal herbs. Congress established the FDA in 1928 in order to rein in charlatans selling unsafe foods and herbal preparations to the unwary public. At the behest of the pharmaceutical industry, Congress passed the Food, Drug, and Cosmetic Act in 1938, which led to the first drug regulations.

In 1962, these regulations were made more strict. In order for any drugs to be sold in the U.S., Congress mandated that drug companies be required to demonstrate a drug's effectiveness and safety. No distinctions were made between new drugs and drugs already on the market.

However, in order to avoid spending millions of dollars to study drugs that had already been safely used for years, the FDA set up oversight panels to review the safety and effectiveness of commonly used ingredients in over-the-counter (OTC) drugs. These panels began in 1972 and completed their work in 1985. They limited their reviews to only products submitted by manufacturing companies. Hundreds of other products were not considered and were left out. Most medicinal plants and herbs were not included in these FDA reports.[15]

The Dietary Supplement Health and Education Act was passed by Congress in 1994. This law stipulates that companies that market herbal medicines in the U.S. may not make medicinal claims about their products unless they prove that these claims are valid. To date, few such studies have been done and very few claims have been approved. This is why most herbs marketed in the U.S. are sold as nutritional supplements. No medicinal claims are made.

In the meantime, the FDA has declined requests by representatives of the herbal industry to reopen the review process that was halted in 1985. Today there is comparatively little publicly funded research and informational support available about plant medicines in the U.S. Because of this, the United States is behind other countries in clinical knowledge on how herbal medicines can be used against infections.

Herbal medicine in Europe

In contrast to the United States, both the French and the German governments give official recognition to natural plant medicines and sanction their use in health care. In Germany, only medical doctors or trained naturopathic physicians are allowed to prescribe essential oils and herbs. Nurses and therapists may dispense essential oils, but only under a doctor's direction. In France, many trained medical doctors use natural plant medicines with their patients.

In Germany as well as France, important milestones have been reached that advance plant medicine to levels unheard of in the U.S. In 1978, the German government convened a panel of experts, the Commission E, to review the scientific literature about essential oils and herbs. More than 650 medicinal plants were included in these studies. Hundreds of medicinal plants were given a stamp of approval for a wide range of therapeutic applications, and their uses, dosages, and possible side effects were published in official *monographs*, or reports.

In France, important developments took place in the field of aromatherapy. Although essential oils were used since the time of the ancient Egyptians, the French "rediscovered" essential oils in the twentieth century.

Chapter 2
Natural Antibiotics

*"With the recent crisis of AIDS, cholera, the increased
incidence and spread of malaria, the possible re-emergence of
smallpox and the appearance of alarming mutant viruses,
the world is now starting to take a more serious look at
herbalism...research into plant medicine is now taking place
more than ever before in the history of medicine."*
—Barbara Hey

In 1928, a French perfumer named Rene-Maurice Gattefosse accidentally burned his hand. The hand became infected and produced a foul odor. Thinking that it could mask the unpleasant odor, Gattefosse applied Lavender essential oil to his wound. To his surprise, he noticed that after a few days his wound began to heal. The odor disappeared and there was no pain, blistering, or scarring left on his hand. Gattefosse hypothesized that although the essential oil was externally applied, it must have been able to penetrate the skin and affect the body internally. This would explain its healing effects.

Gattefosse spent the next years in experimentation and research. He used the scientific method, focusing on the pharmacological effects of essential oils. Because essential oils have aromatic properties, he called this new discipline "aromatherapy."

Following the publication of Gattefosse's research, aromatherapy knowledge gradually spread in France. Initially, aromatherapy was not considered a separate discipline from medicine. French medical researchers were primarily interested in studying the constituents of essential oils to determine their properties and medicinal effects. Jean Valnet, a medical doctor based in Paris, was among those who began experimenting with essential oils. He eventually began treating patients with essential oils and used them for a wide range of conditions:

"As a surgeon during World War II, Dr. Jean Valnet used
essential oils for the treatment of both physical and

psychiatric disorders, sometimes administering them by oral means, with outstanding success. His method, which involved testing specific oils on cultured bacteria taken from the site of the infection, was used not only to ascertain the minimum dosage levels required for various essential oils, but also to find which oils were best suited to treating a particular infection…the results often showed that several oils had similar effects on the same infection."[1]

In 1964, Valnet published a book in France that was widely read and gave great impetus to the medical use of essential oils. In his *The Practice of Aromatherapy*, Valnet reviewed the scientific research concerning the antiseptic actions of essential oils.

Essential oil science

The first early studies on essential oils were done by Chamberland in 1887. Chamberland studied the antibacterial properties of the vapor of Oregano, Cinnamon, Angelica, and Geranium essential oils, and he tested these against certain disease-causing illnesses. He found that essential oils were effective against *Meningococcus*, *Staphylococcus*, and the *Typhus* bacillus; in vapor form they were less effective against Diphtheria germs and not at all effective against Anthrax spores.

In 1918, Cavell conducted experiments with microbic cultures found in sewage water. He observed that essential oils even in dilute amounts showed antiseptic action.[2] For every thousand parts of microbic culture, only minute amounts of essential oils were needed to effectively neutralize microbes found in the water.

Cavell's results were later duplicated by other researchers, but using different types of cultures. Clove Bud essential oil was found to kill the Tuberculosis bacillus at the rate of one part to six thousand; Thyme essential oil was effective as a half-percent solution against the Typhus bacillus as well as the Shiga's bacillus—the bacillus that causes epidemic dysentery.[3]

In the 1930's, Belgian researchers experimented with essential oils against different types of bacterial cultures. Using a 5% solution of essential oil constituents (Geraniol, Borneol, and Cypress), they tested the solution against *Staphylococcus aureus, Typhus bacillus, Colon bacillus, bacillus Foecalis alcaligene,* and *Bacillus subtilis.* Of the different bacterial cultures tested, all except *Bacillus subtilis* were effectively sterilized when the solution was administered at room temperature.

These findings prompted the Belgian researchers to conduct further experiments, both on animals and humans, using intravenous injections. To assure sterility, the essential oils were first heated to 105° C and kept at this temperature for 20 minutes before they were administered. But even after heating, the essential oils retained their bactericidal properties, and the injections caused no painful reactions or side effects in either animal or human subjects.

In the 1960s, studies were done by Professor Griffon on the bacterial purification of room air. Griffon was then the Director of the French Police Toxicology Laboratory and also a member of the Higher Council for Hygiene in France. Griffon studied the virulence of microscopic germs present in the air before and after exposure to essential oils.

When petri dishes containing a growing nutrient were set out at ground level in a room and allowed to stand undisturbed, microscopic flora, found in the air, settled in the dishes and soon began to grow. After just 15 minutes, researchers already found 62 colonies growing in the culture! These included eight mold colonies and six colonies of *Staphylococci* bacteria. After 24 hours, 210 colonies of microscopic flora were found, including 12 mold cultures and eight cultures of *Staphylococci!*

Next, the room was disinfected using an air spray containing essential oils. Only fifteen minutes after spraying, the cultures growing in the dishes had been reduced to 14, including only four mold cultures and no *Staphylococci!* After thirty minutes in the sprayed room, a few colonies still remained in the petri dishes, but no molds or *Staphylococci* cultures were found.

Griffon's study showed that dispersing essential oils into the atmosphere resulted in a marked disinfection of the room air, demonstrated by the rapid reduction in the number of microscopic cultures found in the petri dishes. Some types had completely been destroyed.[4] Valnet, commenting on the work of Griffon, stated that these studies "proved that the disinfection of the air surrounding the patient has a therapeutic [and] preventative effect."[5] He therefore advocated disinfecting the air found in sick rooms or clinics with essential oils, especially for childhood illnesses such as colds, nasal catarrh, influenza, and whooping cough; and for adult illnesses such as influenza, TB, and pneumonia.

Modern French research

In the 1970s, French medical doctors Jean Claude Lapraz and Christian Duraffourd, students of Valnet, began performing clinical trials and researching effective methods of combating infections. Eventually, they documented over 3,000 clinical cases regarding the effects of essential oils with a wide variety of infectious illnesses. They gave consideration not only to the antibiotic properties of essential oils, but also to the oils' ability to create equilibrium in the nervous and the endocrine system. They believed that by improving the body's equilibrium and by balancing the body's internal chemistry (the biological terrain), patients could resist infections successfully.

Lapraz and Duraffourd have many publications to their credit. Their book *ABC De La Phytotherapie Dans Les Maladies Infectieuses* [loosely translated, "The ABCs of Phytotherapy in Infectious Illnesses], first published in France in 1978, contains an overview of their theoretical approach and also gives examples of how particular infections are treated using essential oils and herbal tinctures.[6]

In 1979, Dr. Paul Belaiche, another French doctor affiliated with the Phytotherapy Department at the University of Paris, published a three-volume study on the clinical uses of aromatherapy for treating infectious diseases. In these volumes he introduced what is known as *The Aromatic Index*. This index summarizes the results of more than 20 years of studies on the anti-infectious properties of essential oils.[7] 42 essential oils were studied against 12 of the most common pathogenic microorganisms, including *E. coli*, two different strains of *Staphylococcus*, *Pneumococcus*, and *Streptococcus B*. The index divides the essential oils into three categories, according to their overall effectiveness against disease-causing germs.

In the first group, Belaiche listed the essential oils that showed the greatest consistency and strength against the microorganisms tested. These included Oregano, Savory, Cinnamon Bark, Thyme, and Clove

Bud essential oils. He later added Tea Tree essential oil to this group, after the anti-infectious properties of tea tree were better known.

In the second group, Belaiche listed essential oils of average effectiveness. This list included Cajeput, Myrtle, Eucalyptus, Pine Needle, Lavender, Tarragon, and Niaouli.

The remaining essential oils in Belaiche's study did not appear to have a direct inhibitory effect on infectious microbes. In spite of these findings, many aromatherapists believe that other essential oils, including those not studied by Belaiche, have antibiotic effects. They lack antiseptic properties, but cure infections by working indirectly on the body. Research shows that many different essential oils have been proven effective against infections—in the laboratory as well as under clinical conditions.

Medical aromatherapy today

Because of their clinical success in treating patients, Duraffourd and Lapraz have been very active in promulgating medical aromatherapy worldwide. They were instrumental in organizing the first International Phytotherapy Conference, which was held in Tunisia in May of 1993. Among the countries represented at the conference were the United States, China, India, Turkey, Greece, Egypt, Algeria, Mexico, Madagascar, Morocco and Senegal. The purpose of the conference was to assess the status of plant medicine in various countries and to report research. The papers presented at this conference were later published.[8]

At this conference, Duraffourd and Lapraz presented several papers giving their own clinical studies. They largely duplicated the results reported earlier by Dr. Paul Belaiche in 1979. Following Belaiche's example, Duraffourd and Lapraz tested 48 essential oils. The illnesses tested against included infections of the respiratory organs, the digestive tract, the urinary tract, and the male and female genitals. As Belaiche had done, they developed a method for quantitatively evaluating the overall bactericidal effectiveness of essential oils.

When their work was completed, they listed the essential oils of Oregano, Cinnamon Bark, Thyme, Clove Bud, Cajeput, Savory, Lavender, Pine Needles, Myrtle, Geranium, and Eucalyptus as being the most anti-infectious essential oils.[9] These results were similar to those of Belaiche. They agreed that Oregano, Cinnamon Bark, Thyme, and Clove

Bud essential oils were the strongest, most consistently effective antibiotic essential oils against different types of infectious illnesses.

A closer look at antibiotic essential oils

Oregano (*Oreganum vulgare*) should not be confused with the kitchen spice or the ingredient commonly found on pizza. Oregano essential oil is obtained from a wild plant variety found in Spain. The plant is rich in carvacrol, which is a natural bactericide. Oregano essential oil also has antiviral and antifungal properties.

Dr. Cass Ingram says that Oregano essential oil is "the Rolls Royce of all natural antiseptics."[10] Dr. Kurt Schnaubelt writes that essential oil of Oregano is "aromatherapy's heavy artillery" against bacterial infections.[11] Oregano has a pale, brown-yellowish color and its odor resembles camphor. It has a wide range of medical uses. Most commonly, it is used for viral infections such as a cold, flu, bronchitis, or pneumonia. It is effective for all respiratory conditions, including pulmonary tuberculosis and whooping cough. Applied to the skin, the oil can be used against chronic fungal infections, such as fungal nail infection and athlete's foot.

Cinnamon Bark (*Cinnamomum zeylanicum*) is one of the oldest known spices. The tree is cultivated in India, Sri Lanka, Mauritius, and the Seychelles. The bark is removed from 6–8 year old trees, then cut into strips and left to dry in the sun. The essential oil is steam-distilled from the sun-dried bark.

Cinnamon Bark essential oil is an effective stimulant for the circulatory system and an analgesic for treating muscle aches and pain. It has strong antiviral, antifungal, and antibacterial properties due to its main ingredient, cinnamaldehyde. In their clinical studies, Lapraz and Duraffourd successfully used Cinnamon Bark essential oils to treat skin infections, infections of the respiratory system, digestive tract infections, and foremost, bacterial bladder infections.[12] Used internally, Cinnamon Bark essential oil stimulates secretions of the digestive system.[13]

Thyme (*Thyme serpyllum*) is a valuable natural disinfectant. Thyme is extensively used commercially in mouthwashes, gargles, toothpastes, cough drops, after shave lotion, soap, and toiletries.[14] The essential oil is obtained either from the fresh herb—a small, 18-inch high evergreen shrub found in the Mediterranean—or from the partly dried leaves and flowering tops.

Due to its antiseptic properties, Thyme essential oil may be used to treat infections in all body systems, especially the respiratory system. It is excellent for bronchitis, coughs, colds, and flu. It expels worms from the digestive tract. Thyme essential oil is warming, stimulating, and fortifying; it stimulates the brain, increases metabolism, and aids the nervous system in coping with stress.

Clove Bud (*Syzygium aromaticum*) is an essential oil with strong antiviral, antiseptic, and antibacterial properties. During the sixteenth century, cloves were used with pomanders to ward off the plague. Another traditional use of cloves is as a toothache remedy. "A sucked clove has helped numb a toothache for centuries."[15] Cloves are native to the Mollucan islands of Indonesia; now they are cultivated in many tropical countries.

Clove Bud essential oil is an analgesic used to alleviate skeletal and muscle pain. Taken internally in small doses, it can remove intestinal parasites, worms, and their eggs. Diluted Clove Bud essential oil can be used for skin and hair conditions such as measles, scabies, athlete's foot and lice.

Tea tree (*Melaleuca alternifolia*) and Eucalyptus (*Eucalyptus globulus*) are essential oils from Australia. They are both members of the Myrtaceae plant family. The aboriginal people of Australia were familiar with their use, and early European settlers learned about them from the natives. During colonial times, Tea Tree essential oil was considered a "bush remedy" for all types of infection. Beginning in the 1920s, Tea Tree oil began to attract the attention of Australian scientists and researchers. Its reputation spread, and soon it was considered a "miracle remedy." Tea Tree oil was issued to Australian soldiers during World War II in their first aid kits. Today, both Tea Tree and Eucalyptus essential oils are widely used for their bactericidal, antifungal, and antiviral properties.[16]

Many research studies have been done that confirm Tea Tree oil's traditional use as an antiseptic. At the recent 69th Annual Meeting of the American Academy of Orthopaedic Surgeons held in Texas on February 14th and 15th, 2002, two surgeons reported that two essential oils— Eucalyptus and Tea Tree—were found surprisingly effective at treating *Staphylococcus aureus* skin infections.

In a 25-patient study, an antibacterial wash derived from these essential oils was applied to infected skin wounds. In 19 cases, the infections resolved without the use of antibiotics, while three patients required antibiotic treatment. These doctors are now continuing their studies by spraying aerosolized versions of their compound in laboratory studies of tuberculosis. Initial reports indicate that they are very effective against TB.[17]

Antibiotic herbs

Essential oils are not the only plant medicines with antibiotic properties. In addition to essential oils, the doctors in France also use antibiotic herbal tinctures to fight infections. When caring for patients with infectious illnesses such as bronchitis, colitis, bladder infection, and vaginitis, they combine different essential oils and herbs, using both types of plant medicines simultaneously.

According to Rita Elkins, a Master Herbalist and a published author in the field of herbal medicine, most plant remedies are more effective when you use two or more together rather than one alone, because one supplements the other.[18] Combining different plant medicines together lessens the chance that a particular germ or microbe can develop resistance to the medicine, and increases the chances for success in treatment.

The herbs chosen are sometimes well-known natural antibiotics, such as Echinacea, Garlic, and Goldenseal. At other times, herbal tinctures are chosen for their specific medicinal effects or for their general ability to support the body. There are many herbal tinctures. In this section, I will mention only a few.

Garlic (*Allium sativum*) has been called "the wonder herb."[19] It is one of the world's oldest herbal medicines, and one of the best. In the last 30 years, more than 2,000 scientific studies have been done on garlic.

A member of the Lily family, Garlic contains more than 200 different chemical compounds.[20] The antibiotic properties of Garlic come from allicin and ajoene, which are substances containing sulphur. One milligram of allicin is estimated to equal fifteen standard units of penicillin. During World War II, when Russian doctors ran out of conventional medical supplies, they relied on Garlic to treat the wounded. This is why Garlic is sometimes called the "Russian penicillin."

Goldenseal (*Hydrastis canadensis*) has been called "a potent antibiotic."[21] Goldenseal is used to fight bacterial infections accompanied by fever and inflammation.

The two active chemical constituents of Goldenseal are berberine and hydrastine. The berberine in Goldenseal kills many of the bacteria that cause diarrhea, including *E. coli*, *Salmonella*, *Shigella*, *Klebsiella*, and *Vibrio cholerae*, which causes cholera.[22] As a natural antibiotic, Goldenseal protects against both gram-positive and gram-negative bacteria, including the bacteria that causes tuberculosis. Goldenseal is also used against the protozoan animals that cause amoebic dysentery (*Entamoeba histolytica*), giardiasis (*Giardia lamblia*), and trichomoniasis (*Trichomonas vaginalis*). As an antifungal agent, Goldenseal is effective against *Candida albicans*.

Bayberry (*Berberis vulgaris*) and Oregon Grape (*Berberis aquifolium*) are herbs that also contain berberine; like Goldenseal, they have antibiotic effects. Laboratory studies confirm that Oregon Grape is as effective a bactericide against strep infections as Goldenseal. Berberine-containing plants have been found to be more potent against malaria-related parasites than the antibiotic tetracycline. Berberine also inhibits cancer cell formation and reduces inflammation.[23]

Herbs used for systemic support

In addition to the herbs already mentioned, there are many other herbs with antibiotic properties. Some herbs are not selected just for their infection fighting abilities, but rather for their specific medicinal effects and because they support the body, either before, during, or after an illness episode. Certain herbs are powerful stimulants for the immune system, others are used to prevent disease, still others are helpful to specific body systems.

Plants that contain antioxidants are disease-preventing plants. Antioxidants prevent or delay oxidation, a chemical reaction that can lead to the build-up of toxins in the body. Antioxidants are found in dark-colored fruits and berries. Examples include blueberries, blackberries, raspberries, cherries, cranberries, red grapes, plums, raisins, and prunes. In herbal medicine the juice or tinctures of these antioxidant plants are often prescribed. Cranberry is used as a preventive for urinary tract infections because certain antioxidant compounds found in Cranberry prevent bacteria from adhering to the bladder.[24]

Immune-stimulating herbs are herbs that stimulate the white blood cells. Examples include Astragalus (*Astragalus membranaceus*), Boneset (*Eupatorium perfoliatum*), and Echinacea (*Echinacea angustifolia* or *Echinacea purpurea*). These herbs are commonly used during viral illnesses because they can shorten the duration of these illnesses.

Calendula (*Calendula officinalis*), Lady's Mantle (*Alchemilla vulgaris*), and Yarrow (*Achillea millefolium*) are traditional female remedies. Calendula is a bacteriostatic, but in addition, it reduces inflammation, controls fevers, and assists with the removal of toxins in swollen lymph glands, especially those of the inguinal region. Lady's Mantle is a tonic that helps regulate the menstrual cycle. Yarrow is an antispasmodic herb that can relax the uterus and relieve menstrual cramps. It is also effectively used to control fevers.

Elderberry (*Sambucus canadensis*) is a useful herb with a variety of medicinal actions. Elderberry acts deeply on pulmonary complaints as well as digestive disorders. It opens the lungs, calms croup, and brings up mucus. For digestive complaints, it is used to stimulate the stomach and bowels. It relaxes and tones the tissues of the digestive tract and is effective in reducing colic, bloating, gas, and indigestion. During fevers, Elderberry opens the pores of the skin and induces sweating. Recent scientific studies indicate Elderberry's ability to shorten the duration of viral illnesses.[25]

Good news

Most health care practitioners are very intelligent and open to learning. For the most part, they are somewhat aware about plant medicines and other natural forms of healing. But they are often unsure about what products they can safely recommend to their patients, and how to use them. Health practitioners will use products they believe in. They will use products if they are of good quality and if they work. Doctors cannot afford to have their names linked with remedies that produce uncertain results.

In the United States, the plant medicine market is now worth more than \$4.5 billion per year. More than 800 companies are involved in producing medicinal plant products. According to one group of analysts familiar with this industry, the problem is not a lack of financial success. Rather, there is a problem with product quality and reliability. They ask, "These products are great for business, but are they good for what ails us?"[26]

In a 1998 study by the Consumer Safety Symposium on Dietary Supplements and Herbs, a survey was completed on St. John's Wort, one of the most popular medicinal plants in North America. The survey "showed a 17-fold difference in the concentration of 'active' constituents in commercial preparations of St. John's Wort." [27]

What this demonstrates is that St. John's Wort purchased from one company may not be comparable to St. John's Wort purchased from another company. One product may have excellent medicinal effects, the other may not be as effective. Writing in the New England Journal of Medicine, Marcia Angell and Jerome Kassirer explain the crux of the problem:

> "In response to the lobbying efforts of the multi-billion dollar dietary supplement industry, Congress in 1994 exempted their products from FDA regulation...Since then these products have flooded the market, subject only to the scruples of their manufacturers. They may contain the substances listed on the label in the amounts claimed, but they need not, and there is no one to prevent their sale if they don't. In an analysis of ginseng products, for example, the amount of active ingredient in each pill varied by as much as a factor of 10 among the brands that were labeled as containing the same amount. Some brands contained none at all...the only legal requirement in the sale of such products is that they not be promoted as preventing or treating disease. To comply with that stipulation, their labeling has risen to an art form of doublespeak." [28]

These kinds of variations in product quality and the fact that label information may be inaccurate or misleading place a heavy burden on both health care practitioners and consumers. Under these circumstances, it is difficult to know if a company's claims are true or if their products will actually produce results.

The adulteration of essential oils

Essential oils are especially vulnerable to adulteration. As we discussed in Chapter 1, the world today is divided into two markets:

commercial essential oils are used by the flavor and fragrance industry and medicinal essential oils which are used by people who are interested in health care. The commercial market consumes 90 percent of the world's essential oils. Essential oils are redistilled, blended with additives and sweeteners in the manufacturing of lotions, skin treatments, toothpaste, and other personal care items. Essential oils are also used commercially in cola drinks, candies, cereals, chewing gum, and foods.

The market for medicinal essential oils is small, but the quality standards for medicinal essential oils are much more strict. For health and healing, medicinal essential oils must be raw, unaltered, and genuine. They must be single species essential oils, and they should be used as close to their natural state as possible. The key constituents present must meet medicinal levels in order to be effective.

The quality of essential oils is determined by plant quality, growing conditions, whether the plants have been properly harvested and distilled, how they are stored, and what happens to them after they reach the distributor or manufacturer.

As a consumer of essential oils, it can be challenging to determine if the essential oils offered for sale are therapeutically effective. Unfortunately, labeling practices are sometimes misleading. Here are some examples:

- "Pure" essential oils—In the U.S., "pure" has no legal meaning and can be applied to anything. For example, "pure" can mean part essential oil and part vegetable oil.

- "Extended" essential oils—These are oils that have been diluted with a cheaper mixing oil or synthetic filler. They can also be labeled as "pure."

- "Co-distilled" essential oils—Oils created by adding an essential oil to other plant material to produce one single oil.

- "Rectified" or "redistilled" essential oils—Oils that have had natural components removed from them, especially components that are considered undesirable, such as terpenes or coumarins.

- "Folded" essential oils—Oils that have been redistilled a number of times to make their scent more attractive.

- "Reconstituted" essential oils—Oils that have had natural or synthetic chemicals added to them.

Some companies market oils that have been redistilled to enhance their fragrance, or their essential oils have been diluted with inexpensive vegetable oils and other additives. The average customer will not detect this manipulation.

The only certain way to determine quality is to perform a laboratory analysis using instruments such as the *gas chromatograph* (GC) and *mass spectrometer* (MS). Reputable companies usually have this information available for their customers. The test is commonly known as the GC–MS test.

If you have a concern about where to buy essential oils, please check my internet page **www.healthpracticebooks.com**. Click on "Resources and Links" to find useful information. I don't personally sell essential oils or herbal products on this web page, but I will recommend certain companies who do sell medicinal quality herbal medicines and who provide excellent customer care.

Chemotyped essential oils

A chemotyped oil is an essential oil that has a higher than normal level of one or more of its active ingredients. Chemotyped oils sometimes result from differences in climate, soil, or other natural conditions. *Chemotype* refers to the principal active ingredient that is found in the essential oil of a plant.

There are some important instances where plants of one botanical species will produce essential oils that have different combinations of active ingredients. For example, Wild Rosemary grown near the sea produces constituent levels that may differ from Wild Rosemary grown further inland.

Essential oils are products of nature, and natural variations occur. For the most part, these natural variations do not affect the therapeutic value of essential oils. There are a few exceptions. One variety of essential oil of Basil contains 70% methyl chavicol and 25% linalool. Basil chemotyped linalool contains 50% linalool and 15% methyl chavicol. Both of these oils are produced by the same plant species, but in this case, the variety containing high levels of methyl chavicol should not be used, because it is considered a potential carcinogen.

There are, however, some aromatherapists who espouse the *theory of chemotyping*. This is the notion that the therapeutic effects of essential oils are based solely on the qualities of their principal active ingredients.

For example, the value of Thyme essential oil would be attributed to its principal constituent, thymol, an antimicrobial agent. Likewise, Geranium oil would be considered an effective bactericide because of the properties of its active constituent, geraniol. Those in favor of chemotyped oils claim that they are superior because of the higher percentage of the certain key constituent. And of course, the price is much higher for the chemotyped oil.

This line of reasoning is false and opens the door to the adulteration of essential oils.

In the first place, it is inconsistent with the "Law of All or Nothing." To value an oil only for its most active ingredient negates the work of nature, because "nature does nothing in vain."

In the second place, a series of research studies conducted by Drs. Christian Duraffourd, Dr. Jean–Claude Lapraz, and others on their team disproves the theory of chemotyping.

In these studies, different varieties of essential oils—including their Chemotype—were compared for their effectiveness in clinical trials and also in the laboratory. The results showed that there were few differences among the different essential oil varieties. A chemotyped oil with a higher percentage of an active ingredient was not necessarily superior to an oil with a lower percentage in their antibacterial effects:

> "Reviewing the significance of various compositions of essential oils on their antimicrobial effects, a study was done which compared the effectiveness of different Chemotype of *Thymus vulgaris* on different strains of several microorganisms. The results of this particular study are quite interesting showing that, in many cases, the effectiveness of the Thyme oils have a low phenol content….is the same as that of the high-phenolic type of oils."[29]

The antibiotic effect of essential oils could not be attributed to their principal constituents. It is the essential oil as a totality that has therapeutic value, not the active ingredient in and of itself. Those promoting a chemotyped oil may do so as a marketing ploy to justify higher prices. Or, they may be selling an adulterated product.

Unfortunately, the customer cannot tell if the chemotyped oil is in fact a natural product. Dishonest providers of essential oils have been known to artificially add certain constituents to essential oils and then promote these as chemotyped oils. Unfortunately, these practices destroy consumer confidence and stand in the way of progress. Essential oils and herbal tinctures can be employed with great success to fight infections, but they won't work if they are adulterated or of poor quality.

Chapter 3
Why Use Plant Medicines?

"Modern medicine and science has never proved that herbs do not work, they simply have ignored them. The fad of the hour is to break down substances, not into patterns, but into piles of unrelated constituents. Herbs are not ultimate discrete substances and therefore do not fit this paradigm. They are inconvenient." —Matthew Wood

Just a few years ago, most people believed that the threat of epidemic infectious disease was a thing of the past. Following the introduction of penicillin during World War II, steady progress was made against illnesses such as tuberculosis (TB), malaria, and smallpox. In 1980 authorities announced that they had eradicated smallpox. And as recently as 1996, a joint study by the World Bank/World Health Organization (WHO) projected dramatic reductions in the incidence of infectious diseases.

But now, infectious diseases of all types are suddenly front page news again. How things have changed! The cruel, destructive acts against the Pentagon and the World Trade Centers on September 11, 2001, and the subsequent anthrax attacks suddenly made everyone feel much more vulnerable to the threat of biological warfare. For the first time, we now understand clearly how likely we are to experience such attacks—and how poorly prepared we are to face them!

In addition, the news media increasingly reports on the growing threat of infectious diseases worldwide. Twenty well-known infectious diseases—including TB, malaria, and cholera—have recently reemerged and are spreading globally, often in more virulent forms than before. And, since 1973, at least 30 new, previously unknown disease-causing microbes have been identified. These include HIV, Ebola, Hepatitis C, and Nipa virus, diseases for which no cures are available.[1]

Furthermore, reports about drug-resistant germs are more numerous than ever before. It was recently reported that penicillin has lost its effectiveness against certain strains of pneumonia, meningitis, and gonorrhea. In addition, there is increasing microbial resistance to drugs used to treat HIV/AIDS. According to recent reports, the number of fatalities from HIV/AIDS will likely rise.[2] According to an article in the February 2002 U.S. edition of National Geographic Magazine, "at least 20 major maladies have reemerged in novel, more deadly, or drug-resistant forms in the past 25 years."[3]

With increasing microbial resistance to drugs, the likelihood of a global *pandemic* also increases. "The dramatic increase in drug-resistant microbes, combined with the lag of development of new antibiotics, the rise of megacities with severe health care deficiencies, environmental degradation, and the growing ease and frequency of cross-border movements of people and produce have greatly facilitated the spread of infectious diseases."[4] Because these trends are irreversible, they are likely to continue into the next foreseeable future.

How will we be affected?

The bubonic plague of the 14th century, known as the Black Death, eliminated about one-fourth of Europe's population in a period of only four years. When the Europeans colonized the New World, their diseases wiped out huge numbers of American Indian natives. The last great flu pandemic of 1918–1919 left 20 million dead. Today, with our massive urban populations and close contact between peoples as a result of international travel, the prospect of a new pandemic "is not a matter of if, but when."[5] The problem is so grave that in 1999, the U.S. government's Central Intelligence Agency conducted a study on the global infectious disease threat and its implications to the security of the United States.[6]

The CIA examined major risk factors posed by infectious diseases over the next 20 years and then projected three different scenarios. The first scenario, labeled "steady progress," in the fight against infectious disease, was considered the least likely to occur. In this scenario, economic development and advances in health care would produce a major breakthrough leading to the effective control of disease outbreaks. This scenario was considered unlikely to happen because of global social and economic challenges, the increase in drug-resistant germs, and "because related models have already underestimated the force of major killers such as HIV/AIDS, TB, and malaria."[7]

The second scenario, labeled "progress stymied," was more

pessimistic but also more plausible than the first. Under this scenario, drug-resistant strains of TB, malaria, and other infectious diseases appear more rapidly than new drugs or vaccines, creating widespread havoc. In addition, the incidence of HIV/AIDS increases catastrophically in Latin America, India, China, and the former Soviet Union. Although judged more likely to occur than the first scenario, this second scenario was deemed unlikely because of economic development, international collaboration, and advances in medicine. These trends can slow the spread of at least some of these diseases.

The third and final scenario was labeled "deterioration, then limited improvement." According to CIA estimates, this scenario was most likely to occur, "barring the appearance of a deadly and highly infectious new disease, a catastrophic upward lurch by HIV/AIDS, or the release of a highly contagious biological agent."[8] This scenario foresees a deterioration in world health conditions caused by infectious diseases during the next decade, followed by gradual improvements. These improvements would come about as a result of demographic changes (e.g., a low birth rate), social and economic changes, better surveillance and response systems, and medical advances.

The U.S. poorly prepared to face an epidemic

The findings from the CIA indicate that health conditions will decline before they get better, and the threat from infectious diseases will increase. With our world more and more interdependent, infectious diseases are no longer only a third-world problem, but a problem for all mankind. Infectious diseases were the leading cause of death worldwide during the year 1998, the last year global estimates were available. In the U.S. alone, annual infectious disease-related deaths have nearly doubled since 1980, to some 170,000 deaths annually. Influenza now kills 30,000 Americans each year.[9]

Although the American medical system is excellent in many ways, we cannot rely on this system with blind faith. Drugs and common medical procedures also can cause illness. There are drugs with unwanted secondary effects, surgeries of questionable value, prescription errors, hospital mistakes, and treatments that do not result in a cure. Deaths resulting from the *correct* use of prescription medicines now exceed 100,000 people annually, more than double the rate of deaths resulting from automobile accidents.[10] This year, more than 14,000 people will die as a result of infections *caught in hospitals.*[11]

When faced with illness epidemics or even biological warfare, the U.S. is poorly prepared. Under normal conditions hospitals in many U.S. cities are nearly full, operating at peak capacity. If an epidemic breaks out, doctors, hospitals, and care facilities will be overwhelmed. Civil defense exercises and simulations conducted by various groups show that most hospitals will not be able to deal with a flood of patients should an epidemic, nuclear war, biological or chemical attack occur.[12] Hospitals simply do not have enough beds in emergency rooms or hospital wards to care for thousands of people streaming in for treatment. Patients will be cared for in hotels, armories, or college dormitories, but the level of care provided in those places cannot equal those of hospitals, and the numbers of available trained medical personnel may be insufficient.[13]

A related danger is the time of delay between the outbreak of an epidemic and the government's ability to organize an emergency response. The government depends on reports from doctor's offices and city and county health departments for indications of an unusual outbreak of illness. Many serious illnesses, especially those most apt to be used in biological warfare, have initial symptoms similar to the common cold or flu. People may not recognize those symptoms promptly enough and will try to treat their illness at home. Even if people go to the doctor on time, there may be delays in recognizing and reporting new epidemic outbreaks. Numerous days may be taken up before authorities can determine the extent of the problem. By then it may be too late to save lives—thousands of people could die.

Currently, the U.S. has no reliable system in place for detecting new disease outbreaks and reporting findings. The Center for Disease Control (CDC) is now planning to implement a $90 million Health Alert Network via the internet that will connect local, state, and federal health agencies, *but it could take years before the system is up and running.*[14]

Antibiotics not always available

In an epidemic, health officials rely on stockpiles of vaccines and antibiotic drugs which have been stored away for use in an emergency. In the past year, concerns have been raised about the supply levels of certain of these drugs, most notably anthrax vaccines and inoculations against smallpox. The federal government has negotiated with manufacturers to step up production and increase supplies. No one knows for sure if the levels of supply planned by officials will be sufficient in the event of a national epidemic. Transportation system failure is another cause for concern, and so is the question of whether or not—especially under conditions of quarantine—hospitals and clinics will be able to receive the needed supplies.

Moreover, no one can be sure that the medications stored away will be effective against the particular infectious agents causing the breakout. A good example of this is the viruses that causes influenza. Because they are prone to mutate, influenza viruses continually appear in different forms. A new flu vaccine must be produced every season. In some years, this causes no concern because symptoms are mild. In other years, however, symptoms can be lethal. There were deadly outbreaks of influenza in1918–1919, in 1957–1958, and again in 1968–1969; millions died. An avian flu outbreak in Hong Kong in 1997 cost hundreds of millions of dollars in lost poultry production, commerce, and tourism.[15]

Antimicrobial resistance occurs when a disease-causing germ (bacteria, fungus, parasite, or virus) is no longer affected by a drug that previously was either able to kill it or prevent it from growing. Even among germs that are susceptible to a drug, a small percentage is always naturally resistant. Eventually, this proportion of drug-resistant microbes grows, rendering drugs ineffective.

Germs constantly evolve, developing into new, virulent strains. Because of this, researchers must constantly develop newer and stronger antibiotics. They are becoming increasingly less successful, and often bacteria appear to have the upper hand. Bacterial microbes live everywhere and they reproduce quickly. They can easily share genetic information with each other, and even with cells from a different species. Once a bacteria survives destruction by antibiotics, it can pass the genes of destruction on to other germs. Bacteria seem to be winning the battle against medical science.[16]

> "The growth and intensity of antimicrobial resistance among infectious pathogens increases, due both to pathogen mutation and indiscriminate use of therapeutic drugs…Two-thirds of all oral antibiotics worldwide are

obtained without a prescription and are inappropriately used against diseases such as TB, malaria, pneumonia, and more routine childhood infections. These practices contribute to antimicrobial resistance and the severe, nearly impossible to treat hospital-acquired infections... Some epidemiologists and health experts have even suggested that we may be entering a post-antibiotic era in which antimicrobials, in general, will lose their effectiveness against the most common diseases."[17]

The overuse of antibiotics

One important reason for the increase in antibiotic-resistant strains of bacteria is the widespread misuse of antibiotics. According to various estimates, between 40 and 70% of all antibiotics are prescribed unnecessarily or erroneously. "Many physicians and dentists prescribe antibiotics 'just in case' and as much as 70% of the time these drugs are prescribed wrongly."[18]

In the case of viral infections, antibiotics are often prescribed to prevent a *superinfection*, a new infection caused by an organism different from the one that caused the initial infection. But treating patients with antibiotics to prevent superinfection is unnecessary if essential oils are used. Therefore, one benefit of essential oils and other herbal medicines is that they can reduce our dependence on antibiotics, especially when antibiotics are known not to be effective against viral diseases.

The large-scale use of antibiotics causes microbes to evolve into new forms in order to survive. According to Leon Chaitow, an English naturopath, "the crisis in antibiotic use which has gradually emerged over the past 15 or 20 years or so is only partly the result of misuse or overuse of these potentially life-saving drugs. It is also in large part the natural... outcome of an attack on a life-form which has found ways of protecting itself—by mutation, by natural selection, as well as in-built resistance."[19]

Marc Lappe, author of *When Antibiotics Fail* writes, "We have let our profligate use of antibiotics reshape the evolution of the microbial world and wrest any hope of sage management from us...Resistance to antibiotics has spread to so many different, and such unanticipated types of bacteria, that the only fair appraisal is that we have succeeded in upsetting the balance of nature."[20]

The overuse of antibiotics is not limited to the practice of modern medicine. Antibiotics are found everywhere, even in our food supply; they are added to animal feed to prevent bacterial infections. As in humans, animals exposed to antibiotics on a daily basis can develop antibiotic-resistant strains of bacteria in their bodies. When humans eat their meat without proper cooking, these same antibiotic strains colonize in the human gastrointestinal tract. When a person is exposed to the infectious agents, it is feared that he or she may not be able to resist the new disease because of their presence. Outbreaks of this type have already occurred.[21]

Because germs are increasingly resistant to drugs, even more powerful drugs are required to control them. Stronger drugs cause more side effects, so that drugs today are more dangerous to use than before—and more expensive! This has greatly contributed to today's medical crisis. Many doctors now prescribe additional drugs along with antibiotics, drugs that are needed to control the unwanted side effects from the antibiotic medications. Oftentimes the combination of drugs taken seem overwhelming to the patient and make the patient more sick than the disease that originally caused the problem!

Using antibiotics can lead to further illness

When antibiotics are prescribed, they should be used with care, in strict limits and as intended by the manufacturers of the drugs. Many health care practitioners firmly advocate that antibiotics should be reserved until absolutely necessary, because careless use can depress the immune response and lead to further illness.

Elizabeth Lipski, a board-certified clinical nutritionist and author of several books on digestive health, says that certain portions of our gastrointestinal tract, including the mouth, the small intestine, and the colon, are populated by trillions of "friendly bacteria." There are more than 400 different types, and each type can have many different strains. These friendly flora contribute to our health by increasing our immune competence, our ability to ward off infectious disease. In addition to being our "front line" defense against infections, they eliminate wastes and provide many other health benefits.[22]

When antibiotics are used, the antibiotics kill both harmful and friendly bacteria. As a result, harmful elements such as *Candida albicans* are are no longer held in check. They take over the space vacated by the friendly bacteria, causing many types of chronic illnesses and symptoms.

In addition, antibiotics can cause diarrhea and other disorders of the digestive system. The frequent use of antibiotics is the most common reason why people suffer from intestinal dysbiosis (imbalance of the intestinal flora), *Candida albicans,* and associated yeast infections such as thrush and vaginitis.

Other researchers have also discovered that the use of antibiotics can be linked to chronic illnesses such as asthma and chronic fatigue syndrome.[23] In one study cited, up to 80 percent of patients diagnosed with chronic fatigue had a history of frequent use of antibiotics.[24] Dr. Leon Chaitow, author of *Antibiotic Crisis, Antibiotic Alternatives,* links antibiotic use to health problems including elevated cholesterol levels, menopausal symptoms, osteoporosis, gynecological symptoms, liver disease, irritable bowel or chronic digestive problems, increased risk of bladder infection, and arthritic problems.[25]

How to stay alive around drug resistant germs

In 1995, a meeting was held by the Royal Society of Medicine in London where methods used by French doctors to treat infections were demonstrated. Of great interest to those present was the ability of certain essential oils to clear up infections caused by MRSA.[26] MRSA refers to mecithilin-resistant *Staphylococcus aureus* (mecithilin is an antibiotic used to treat staph infections).

An estimated 80,000 people per year get MRSA infections in the U.S.[27] Up to 90 percent of all MRSA strains are resistant to commonly used antibiotics. Some strains are resistant to almost all antibiotics except to those that are also toxic to the human body.[28]

Patients susceptible to MRSA are those with open wounds (such as bed sores), patients who have tubes inserted into their bodies (such as urinary catheters), the elderly, and those who are very sick or weak. The majority of infections are spread in hospitals, where the death rate among those affected by MRSA has reached 14%.[29]

Drug-resistant Streptococcus Pneumonia Disease (DRSP) is another illness caused by drug-resistant germs. DRSP has been increasing steadily in the U.S. since 1987. Of more than 100,000 hospitalizations per year for pneumonia, 40% are thought to be caused by DRSP.[30] Those most at risk are people in nursing homes, extended-care facilities, child-care centers, or hospitals and clinics. DRSP is spread through person-to-person contact.

Plant medicines are potent germ killers

Essential oils are effective *bactericidals* (they kill bacteria) as well as *bacteriostatics* (they inhibit their growth). One of the main reasons for using essential oils is that *germs can develop a resistance to antibiotic drugs but they cannot develop resistance against essential oils.* Essential oils contain chemical compounds—terpenes, sesquiterpenes, aldehydes, alcohols, and phenols—that are lethal to germs. Essential oils have many such chemical compounds and their composition is complex. They are so numerous that disease-causing microbes cannot form a defense against them.

Tests have been conducted to determine if essential oils are as effective against bacteria as common antibiotics. In one such test, the bacteria *E. coli* and *Staphylococcus aureus* were cultivated in petri dishes. Researchers then applied essential oils and common antibiotics to these cultures, to determine which was more potent. The antibiotics used were penicillin and ampicillin; the essential oils tested were Cinnamon Bark (*Cinnamomum zeylanicum*) and Oregano (*Oreganum vulgare*).

By measuring the "zone of inhibition"—the area free of bacterial growth in each dish after applying the antibiotic agent—researchers could find out which of these agents was most effective. Surprisingly, when essential oils were compared to antibiotics, the results were virtually identical. The measurements showed very little variation. Researchers then concluded that the essential oils were comparable in antimicrobial strength to the antibiotics used in the study.[31]

The Aromatogram

In French medical aromatherapy, doctors use a method called the *aromatogram* to determine which essential oils are best to use in cases of infectious disease. Because aromatherapy is a recognized medical discipline in France, French doctors have access to laboratories and equipment that enable them to effectively fight infectious diseases using a full range of medical procedures.

When a person in France has an infectious illness and seeks care from a doctor trained in plant medicine, the doctor will often first order lab work to be done. In this procedure, a specimen is taken from the patient and cultivated in a round petri dish on a nutrient, such as *agar*. Then a patch of blotter paper, impregnated with an essential oil, is added to the center of the dish. After a period of time, usually 18 to 22 hours, technicians examine the culture to determine the effect of the essential oil on the infectious organism.

This can be determined by the extent to which the bacterial culture grew. The more effective the essential oil, the lower the amount of bacterial growth. The "killing zone" is the area surrounding the essential oil where no bacteria are found. The diameter of this area is measured. A number of different essential oils can be tested to find out which is the most effective against a particular culture. The results are then communicated to the doctor, who uses this information to determine the patient's treatment.

In the United States, an aromatogram is called a *sensitivity test*. A sensitivity test is commonly performed in hospitals to determine the effectiveness of an antibiotic agent. The procedure is the same as in France, except that in the aromatogram, essential oils are used instead of antibiotics.

If you live in the U.S., have an infection, and your health care practitioner is not prepared to provide you with an aromatogram or sensitivity test, perhaps arrangements can be made with a nearby clinic or laboratory. They may not be familiar with essential oils, but they do understand how to test an antibiotic agent.

How plant medicines are different

The word "antibiotic" means "destructive of life." This is exactly what antibiotics do—they kill bacteria, both the good and the bad. But unlike antibiotics, essential oils do more than just kill germs. Essential oils are natural substances. They are not inimical to the body. Essential oils can benefit the body in several important ways:

- Certain essential oils can stimulate the body's immune system into taking action against invading microbes. This makes the body a less hospitable place for germs to live and multiply.

- Essential oils alter the body's chemistry, the pH balance. If the body's chemistry is out of balance (e.g., too acidic or alkaline), other systems in the body become overburdened in the attempt to compensate.

• Essential oils act on the body's governing systems—the endocrine system and the nervous system. These systems control all body functions. When faced with illness or injury, the governing systems act to maintain homeostasis and ensure the body's survival.

Because of these differences in the mechanisms of action, we should expect different results when essential oils are used. Essential oils are very beneficial to health and their beneficial effects are long lasting. This is not the case with antibiotic drugs.

The alternative health care model

Understanding the dangers associated with antibiotics and avoiding their use when possible (and knowing that there are natural medicine alternatives to treat infections), can lead to a new sense of freedom and security when dealing with health problems, especially in these challenging times with the threat of global infectious epidemics hanging overhead. It may be, as Michael Weiner has suggested, that "...the age of antibiotics is fast coming to a close [and]...positive, preventive health is becoming more important."[32]

Alternative health care is an emerging form of medical care that emphasizes treating the whole person, at many different levels simultaneously in order to remove the root causes of disease. This is also called *holistic healing*. While conventional medicine relies on prescription drugs and invasive procedures, alternative medicine tends to give more equal focus to working with the body, stimulating the body to heal itself. In treating infectious diseases, alternative medicine is concerned with the biological terrain (the body's internal chemistry), the immune response, and the "causes and progression of infection."[33]

Whether or not we get sick depends on two factors: the virulence or strength of the disease-causing agent, and the strength of our immune system. Both are important. If the immune system is strong, it can ward off most attacks. A weak immune system may be caused by poor nutrition, too much stress, over-reliance on drugs, and environmental pollution. Herbal medicine can boost the immune response by stimulating the production of certain white blood cells (leukocytes).[34]

In alternative medicine, signs and symptoms of disease are considered indications of underlying imbalances in the body. It is the health practitioner's job to determine what those underlying imbalances are. When these are properly dealt with, patients begin to lead productive lives again. But this is only possible if practitioners and patients are willing to address the root causes of illness as quickly as possible, and begin treatments using natural plant medicines. Plant medicines are the best medicines available to fight infections.

CHAPTER 4
Understanding Infections

"In the holistic view of aromatherapy, miraculous, one-day cures are not the goal, but a support of the body's defense system in achieving a complete healing through reestablished immunocompetence." —Kurt Schnaubelt

All of us have experienced an infection at one time or other. Infections are the most common of human diseases. Getting an infection may not be a pleasant experience, but it is part of a person's normal life experience and not necessarily cause for alarm. The majority of infections are self-limiting. If an infection is allowed to run its course safely, the body develops antibodies that enable it to resist future attacks.

Health problems result when the invading microbes are too strong for the body to mount an effective defense, or when defenses are too low because the immune system has been compromised. If the pathogens are too virulent for the body to handle on its own, the body needs help in order to recover. There are no better remedies to boost immunity and to treat infections than natural plant medicines—essential oils and herbs.

Bacterial infections

Bacteria are primitive, single-cell organisms without a nucleus that produce disease in various ways. They can excrete toxic substances that damage human tissues, they may become parasites within human cells, or they may form colonies in the human body that disrupt normal processes.

Scientists have classified bacteria in several different ways. One way is to classify them by size and shape. *Bacilli* are large, rod-shaped cells found singly or in groups. *Cocci* are large, round bacteria found singly, in pairs, in strings, or in clusters. Some bacteria are classified as *curved* or *spiral rods* because they have curved rods arranged singly or in strands, or they can be classified as large curved or spiral cells or cell colonies.

Some bacteria are called *small bacteria* because they are so small that some of them were once thought to be viruses. Typically, they are round or oval shaped. They can only reproduce in other living cells.

Examples of bacteria include *Pseudomonas aeruginosa*, a rod-shaped bacteria that can be found in water, soil, and vegetation; *Escherichia coli*, an organism found in the intestines of humans and animals; and *Staphylococcus aureus*, a microbe found in the air, in water, in food, and in the bodies of humans and animals.

Bacteria cause common illnesses including abscesses, anthrax, botulism, cholera, conjunctivitis, dental caries, diphtheria, gastroenteritis, gonorrhea, "legionnaires" disease, Lyme disease, meningitis, parrot fever, pneumonia, rheumatic fever, Rocky Mountain spotted fever, syphilis, tetanus, toxic shock syndrome, typhoid fever, and whooping cough. Many of these illnesses are discussed in Chapter 6.

Viral infections

A *virus* is a microscopic, parasitic entity smaller than a cell. It consists of a nucleic acid molecule bound by a protein coat and sometimes a lipoprotein envelope. Viruses are the smallest of all disease-causing microbes. They invade healthy cells and insert their own genetic code into the host cell's genetic code. This causes the cell to produce viral DNA or RNA. They can then produce more virus particles.

Examples of viruses include *Epstein–Barr virus*, *Influenza A, B*, or *C*, and *Herpes simplex* 1 and 2. Among the most common viral infections there are HIV/AIDS, chicken pox, the common cold, fever blisters and herpes, hepatitis, infectious mononucleosis, influenza, measles, mumps, polio, rabies, German measles (rubella), viral encephalitis, and warts.

Antibiotics are usually not effective against viruses, but now scientists are also producing antiviral drugs. They can do that when the chemical structure of the virus is known.

Antiviral drugs do not kill viruses. They inhibit the reproduction of viruses, slowing the disease down. Commonly used antiviral drugs are acyclovir (ACV) for herpes and azidothymidine (AZT) for HIV/AIDS.

Fungal infections

A *fungus* is an organism similar to a plant, but it lacks chlorophyll. For this reason, it cannot produce its own food. It must consume other organisms or act as a parasite. Many fungi attack tissue on or near the skin or in a mucous membrane. Examples include athlete's foot and vaginal yeast infection. Some types of fungi are systemic, spreading throughout the body. *Candida albicans* is a prominent example.

Fungal infections must be treated using an "inside out" approach. The internal body chemistry must be altered at the same time that topical applications are used on the outside of the body.

Infections from parasites, protozoa, or pathogenic animals

A *parasite* is an organism that lives in or on another organism in order to obtain its nutrients. Parasites include *protozoa* (single-cell organisms larger than bacteria) and *pathogenic animals* such as nematodes, insects, worms, flukes, and snails. Parasites infest human fluids and body cavities and can cause disease by infesting cells or directly destroying them. These cause common illnesses including amebiasis and amoebic dysentery, giardiasis, malaria, trichomoniasis, roundworm infestation, pinworms, tapeworms, liver flukes, snail fever, and threadworm infestation.

In natural medicine, essential oils and herbal tinctures are usually taken internally to expel parasites and worms from the body. These are called *anthelminthic* or *vermifuge* essential oils and herbs.

What happens during an infection

There are five basic symptoms that typically emerge during an infection:

- *Dolor* or pain, especially when the infection is confined to a body cavity and pressure builds up, causing pain. The amount of pain you feel depends on the extent and virulence, or strength of the infection.

- *Calor* or heat, as when you develop a fever. Even minor infections can result in an elevated body temperature.

- *Rubor* or redness. The term discoloration is more accurate, because in advanced infections the color to be seen is actually more blue and gray. In some illnesses, such as tuberculosis, the lesions turn white. If the infection is on the skin, as for example from a pin prick, you can sometimes see a red streak from where the prick occurred.

- *Tumor* or swelling. Swelling is usually not evident when the infection is deep within your body, but becomes more apparent near the surface.

- *Functio laesa,* diminished or disordered body function. This depends entirely on the body part affected and on the virulence of the disease.

These symptoms may be confined to a specific area, as in a local infection, or they may be *systemic* (coursing through the whole body), as in a fever.

What makes infections dangerous is that the amount of damage done often seems out of proportion to the extent of the actual injury. Many deaths have followed from seemingly minor occurrences, such as a small laceration or cut, a bone splinter, or an infection from the bristles of a brush.

How infections spread

Because we've all experienced infections, we are well aware that infections can be passed along in many different ways.

Contagious infections spread when pathogenic organisms are expelled from an infected person's lungs, mouth, or nose, becoming airborne. Anytime someone with an infection coughs or sneezes, they expel droplets of infectious material into the air. These settle on our clothing, walls, and floors, from where they can spread to others.

Infections can also be passed along through *contact*, when we kiss someone or eat with utensils handled by someone who has an infection. STDs (sexually transmitted diseases) fall into this category. Drug users risk infections when sharing needles with others.

Some infections are passed along either directly or indirectly through carriers, including household pets, flies, insects, or farm animals. An animal host that spreads infection is called a *vector*.

Infectious organisms can be found in the food we eat or in the water we drink. Salad vegetables may carry bacteria from the soil or from manure used as fertilizer. Canned foods may contain the toxin that causes botulism. The bacteria that cause colds or sore throat are habitually present in our mouths.

Disease germs that cause infections are with us almost all the time. We do not know exactly the conditions or circumstances under which they can suddenly flourish and cause illness. Our ability to ward off infections depends on our *immunocompetence*, or strength of resistance, and also on the virulence of the particular pathogen to which we are exposed.

Certain types of infectious organisms, those that form spores, resist drying out and remain virulent for a very long time. Bacterial spores are difficult to kill because they are highly resistant to heat and require prolonged exposure to high temperatures in order to destroy them. But when transmitted to man, they can flourish, causing considerable damage.

The stages of an infection

Every infectious illness runs its own course, and each stage of illness requires appropriate treatment. An infection usually begins with a *latent period*, or *period of incubation*. During this stage, the body has been exposed to an invading microorganism, and if the body is susceptible, the microbe begins to grow (if the body is not susceptible, the microbe will not be permitted to grow).

During the latency period, there are no illness symptoms. However, it is not unusual for a person to feel a bit weak or run down. You may feel that you're not your usual self, or that your energy is not as vital and strong.

The period of incubation can last hours, days, weeks or months depending on the type of illness involved. Influenza can take days before the onset of symptoms, gonorrhea can take several weeks, and rabies can take up to three months. Some infections, such as hepatitis C, can take years to develop.

If the infection happens to be contagious, the *contagious period* begins during the stage of latency. You can spread the illness to others until the contagious period passes. *Ebola*, a highly contagious and lethal infectious disease that occurs in tropical Africa, is actually difficult to spread person-to-person because the Ebola microbe evolves so rapidly in the host that the contagious period passes rapidly.

At the *onset of symptoms*, or *eruption*, the body's normal defense mechanisms kick in and the typical infection symptoms (described above) manifest themselves. This is when many patients first see a doctor to find out what type of infection is involved and what treatment measures are needed. In the case of a sore throat, doctors may take a throat culture to find out if you have a bacterial infection. If the answer is positive, they may then prescribe antibiotics to treat the infection.

The *acme* is the period of greatest intensity during the course of disease. Illness symptoms are the most stressful and severe. Essential oils and herbals are very useful during this time to relieve symptoms, but if any of the following occur, you should seek immediate medical care:

- Abdominal pain accompanied by continuous vomiting
- Temperatures higher than 102° Fahrenheit in adults or 103° Fahrenheit in children
- Seizures
- Bloody vomiting or diarrhea, if either lasts more than 24 hours in adults or 12 hours in children
- Difficulty breathing or any other type of trouble with an organ or system
- A stiff neck (a neck that is painful to move) accompanied by flu-like symptoms
- An eye infection
- Severe pain when urinating, accompanied by pain in the back or flank
- Rashes, if they look like small bleeding spots beneath the skin, and are accompanied by high fever or sleepiness, or if they occur inside the eye or mouth

Under normal circumstances the infectious illness runs its course and symptoms gradually improve. After a period of bed rest, the patient begins to feel better. A *period of convalescence* then follows which can last several weeks or months. Patients often discontinue their therapeutic treatments during this time, but this is a mistake. It is important to support the body during the time of recovery, and natural plant medicines are excellent to use.

Although most infectious illnesses are self-limiting, there are often times when complications develop and patients get worse instead of better. If the immune system has been compromised, bacteria, viruses or other microbes may cause superinfections. These are new infections usually unrelated to the original microorganism that first caused the illness. Complications can lead to rapidly deteriorating health. Doctors may choose to administer a round of antibiotic drugs, but in the case of viral illnesses or illnesses caused by drug-resistant germs, these will not be effective.

Chronic infections are recurring illnesses where the illness itself has become a way of life for the patient. Chronic infections are characterized by periods of relative inactivity which then alternate with periods of illness. If a patient has a chronic infection, the immune system is not working as it should. The frequent and continual use of antibiotic drugs, over-the-counter remedies, lack of exercise, a poor diet, exposure to harmful chemicals in our food and personal care products, pollution, stress, or the presence of parasites and worms in our bodies—all contribute to a low immune response and chronic infections.

An *allergy* is chronic illness characterized by an abnormal reaction of the body against certain substances, such as exhaust fumes, petrochemicals, pollens, or food. The immune system identifies these substances as dangerous invaders and activates antibodies against them. An allergy begins when the body is exposed to the offending substance and becomes sensitized. There are no symptoms at the time, but subsequent exposures produce antibodies and symptoms.

Allergies are representative of a class of diseases called *autoimmune disorders*. Although autoimmune disorders are not infections, both types of illness provoke a defensive reaction indicating that the immune system has been compromised.

How immunity works

The immune system is the body's safety net. Every day, potentially harmful bacteria, viruses, and other pathogens invade our bodies. We are protected from these pathogens by the body's remarkable defenses. Whether or not we get sick depends on how strong these defenses are.

The lymphatic system is important to understand how immunity works. The lymphatic system transports *lymph*, a clear, colorless liquid, to all parts of the body. The lymphatic system resembles the blood circulatory system because it is composed of a network of porous lymphatic vessels that are similar to arteries. However, unlike the blood circulatory system, the lymphatic system has no pump like the heart to keep the lymph flowing.

This is one reason why physical exercise is so important to building a strong immune system.[1] During exercise, muscles contract and the rate of breathing increases. These help move lymph throughout the body. The lymphatic system relies on exercise to maintain the flow of lymph. People who exercise regularly are less likely to have colds and flu than people who lead sedentary life styles.

Lymph nodes are temporary collection places located in clusters along the pathways of the lymphatic system. There are hundreds of lymph nodes scattered throughout the body. Some of these nodes may be as small as the head of a pin, others may be as large as a lima bean.

Although there are a few single nodes, most lymph nodes are grouped in clusters. For example, there are clusters of lymph nodes in the region of the neck below the jaw. As a result of a tooth infection, or during a sore throat, these nodes swell. The swelling is caused by the accumulation of toxins. As the lymph is filtered, special white blood cells called *macrophages* remove bacteria and other foreign matter. The swollen nodes indicate that the lymph

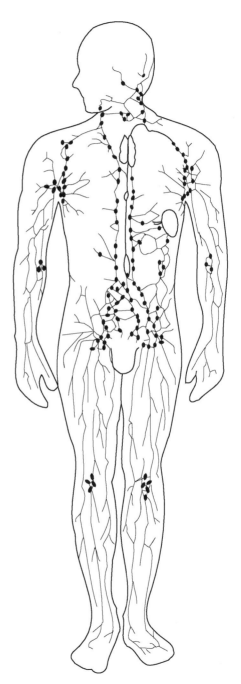

Dots indicate lymph node clusters.

system is working to overpower invading bacteria and other germs.

Defense against an infection is accomplished through *biological filtration*. Special defensive cells called *phagocytic cells* alter the content of the lymph fluid, preventing infections from spreading. When passing through the node, lymph is filtered so that harmful bacteria or other pathogens are removed and prevented from entering the bloodstream and circulating all over the body.

Knowing where lymph nodes are located can be important. Review the figure on the previous page to see where lymph nodes are clustered. Lymph nodes are most easily noticed in the armpits, the groin, the tonsils, the throat, behind joints such as the knee, at the base of the lungs, and in the abdomen. Watch for swelling and tenderness in the lymph nodes for clues that the body may be fighting an infection. When the infection has run its course, the lymph nodes return to their normal size.

If you have swollen lymph nodes that occur without evidence of an infection, or if the swelling persists after the infection has run its course, you should consult with a physician.

The immune system

The *immune system* enables our body to resist infections. The skin and the mucous membranes are mechanical barriers to prevent entry of bacteria, harmful chemicals and toxins, and other substances into the body. Tears and mucus confer general protection rather than protection from specific kinds of invading cells and chemicals.

The body's *inflammatory response* is a non-specific response that happens frequently. Inflammation is characterized by heat, redness, pain and swelling. These signs of inflammation are caused by increased blood flow and permeability in the affected region. Such changes help the white blood cells reach the general area and enter the infected tissue.

Specific immunity confers very specific protection against certain types of invading bacteria. Using memory, the body recognizes specific pathogens and mounts a defense against them. The first time the body is attacked, disease symptoms emerge as the body fights the invasion. When the body is exposed a second time, no symptoms occur because the invading organism is destroyed quickly—the person is said to be immune. Immunity to one type of disease-causing bacteria or virus does not protect the body against others. Immunity can be very selective.

Immunity can be inherited. Some people are not susceptible to certain illnesses because of inherited immunity. A nursing mother can also temporarily pass immunity on to her child through the antibodies found in the mother's milk. This is one reason why breast feeding is beneficial for a young child.

Immunity can also be acquired, either through natural exposure or through immunization.

Immune system cells

The immune system consists of billions of cells. Among these are many different types of immune system cells. The most important immune system cells are called *phagocytes* and *lymphocytes*.

Phagocytes are white blood cells derived from bone marrow. Once in the blood stream, they migrate out of the blood and into the tissues in response to an infection. Two kinds of phagocytes are *neutrophils* and *monocytes*. Neutrophils perform their job and then leave the tissue area where they are. Monocytes stay in the tissue area and develop into specialized phagocyte cells called macrophages. Macrophages "wander" through the tissues to engulf bacteria and other toxins wherever they find them. Certain types of macrophages become residents of certain organs. Macrophages can be found in the liver, the spleen, the lymph nodes, and on the lining membranes of the abdominal and thoracic cavities.

Lymphocytes are the body's most numerous immune system cells. They circulate in the body's fluids, searching for any invading cells that may have entered. Lymphocytes are found throughout the body, but are especially densely populated in the lymph nodes and other lymphatic tissues, the thymus gland, the spleen, and the liver.

There are two major types of lymphocytes: *B-cells* and *T-cells*. B-cells originate in the bone marrow and then migrate to the lymph nodes as immature cells. When they come into contact with antigens, they divide repeatedly. They form *plasma cells*, which secrete antibodies into the blood, and *memory cells*, which are stored in the lymph nodes.

Antibodies are protein compounds normally found in the human body. When the body is invaded, antibodies bind with *antigens* that are found on the surface of the invading germ. Antigens are then changed so that they cannot harm the body. A series of reactions takes place that inactivates or kills the invading cells. When the body is exposed to a particular antigen, the memory cells recognize the antigen and become plasma cells, secreting antibodies into the blood.

Like B-cells, T-cells also originate from stem cells in the bone marrow. A few months before birth and for a short period of time after birth, they migrate to the thymus to develop, and then migrate to the lymph nodes. When an antigen binds to the T-cells' surface proteins, the cells develop into fully sensitized T-cells.

Instead of producing antibodies to fight infections, T-cells destroy microbes. They kill invaders by releasing a substance that poisons them. T-cells also release chemicals that attract macrophages to the area of infection and activate them so they can kill the foreign cells. Certain types of T-cells also signal the brain to increase body temperature so that the immune system can be fully mobilized.

Detoxification

Besides the immune system itself, there are other systems in the body that play a crucial role in maintaining good immune health. These are known as the *organs of detoxification*. The body's major organs of detoxification include the liver, the kidneys, the large intestine, the lungs, and the skin.

The *liver* is the body's largest internal organ. It plays a crucial role in more than 500 different body functions. The liver filters blood and transforms toxins so that they can be eliminated from the body. There are many toxins that can damage the liver. These include alcohol, drugs, pesticides, food additives, prescription drugs, and heavy metals.

When the liver is stressed, many different types of physical and emotional symptoms emerge. These including fatigue, allergies, PMS, headaches, constipation, hypoglycemia, "fuzzy thinking," and poor concentration.

The *kidneys* receive the toxins that the liver has broken down into less harmful substances. They then send them out of the body in the form of urine. The kidneys play a crucial role in maintaining the body's balance of fluids. If the kidneys are stressed and not working efficiently, there may be problems eliminating excess water and mineral salts. This increases blood volume, and forces the heart to work harder than normally needed.

Another important organ of detoxification is the *large intestine*. The large intestine is the pathway for eliminating solid wastes from the body. Food not absorbed into the body in the small intestines enters the large intestine and moves through the colon into the rectum, where it is expelled in bowel movements. Improper elimination is caused by problems such as a lack of fiber in the diet or a low amount of water in the colon. Unless these problems are corrected, inflammation, food allergies, and other health problems result.

The *lungs* bring oxygen to all parts of the body and they also expel poisonous carbon dioxide gases. Lungs are lined with mucous membranes that warm the air as it enters the body. Oxygen is then carried on red blood cells from the lungs to the tissues and cells. Oxygen is necessary for every biochemical process, and when oxygen is not available, cells begin to die. In order for the body to burn fat and produce energy, oxygen must be present. Oxygen deficiency results in a weakened immune system that can lead to viral problems, toxic build-up in the blood, and premature aging.

Carbon dioxide is a waste product produced by the cells when nutrients are broken down. People who do not breathe properly risk leaving carbon dioxide residues in the body. This can result in fatigue and other characteristic symptoms of toxic load.

Environmental toxins such as smog, exhaust fumes, industrial pollutants, and cigarette smoke can impair lung function. Lung congestion can also result from excess food intake or eating too many mucus-forming foods, such as dairy products or products made with flour and sugar.

The *skin* is the largest organ of the body. In adults, the skin weighs 20 pounds or more. It accounts for about 16% of total body weight, and is the body's heaviest organ. One square inch of skin includes:

- 500 sweat glands
- 1,000 nerve endings
- Yards of tiny blood vessels
- Nearly 100 oil or sebaceous glands
- 150 sensors for pressure
- 75 sensors for heat
- 10 sensors for cold
- Millions of cells

The condition of the skin mirrors the health of the body. The skin is an important organ of elimination, and for this reason the skin is sometimes called "the third kidney." Toxins eliminated by the skin through sweating include heavy metals, drugs, pesticides, and other environmental pollutants. If the skin is not efficient in expelling wastes, other organs of elimination, such as the lung, the kidneys, the liver, and the colon are burdened with excess toxins. Conversely, if the large intestine, kidneys, or liver are not adequately detoxifying the body and disposing of wastes, the burden falls to the skin. Acne, boils, skin rashes and other eruptions on the skin are signals that something is amiss in the internal workings of the body's detoxification system.

Toxic load

When there is an excessive build-up of toxins in the body, the body begins to suffer from *toxic load*. Under toxic load, the organs of detoxification become overwhelmed and cannot perform their duties as intended. When toxins are inefficiently removed from the body, body processes stagnate and organ function diminishes. The result is a poor immune system.

Although many different toxins can affect the body, they are easier to understand if they are broken down and classified into two groups:

- *Endotoxins* are wastes that build up inside our body, the by-products from the body's metabolism. Examples of endotoxins are nitrogen wastes (urea) that build up in the body when proteins are digested, excess carbon dioxide that circulates in the bloodstream due to poor circulation, and the wastes produced by intestinal bacteria, parasites, and worms—substances that must be eliminated in order for the body to remain healthy.

- *Exotoxins* enter the body from the outside by inhalation, ingestion, or physical contact.

We are exposed to these toxins by environmental pollution and because the foods they eat and the products they use contain many harmful chemicals. Of the more than 75,000 commercial chemicals in common use today, only 3% have been tested for safety.[2] Among the unsafe chemicals found in products are chemicals that the government does not regulate. In other instances, unsafe chemicals are allowed because occasional exposure causes no lasting harm. But long-term, daily use of chemicals can result in a toxic build-up in the body that can be very harmful.

Common chemicals that are consumed include ingredients such as sodium lauryl sulfate (SLS), diethanolamine (DEA), triethanolamine (TEA), propylene glycol, fluoride, and alcohol. These are found in common personal care products such as shampoo, lotions, toothpaste, and mouthwash. Dr. Samuel Epstein, M.D., author of *The Safe Shopper's Bible* and *The Politics of Cancer Revisited*, has identified these chemicals as known or potential carcinogens.[3]

How infections develop

Infections commonly develop along the body's detoxification pathways as body processes stagnate. The body eliminates toxins through the organs of detoxification, but if these are too stressed the body finds other ways of handling them. Toxins may be stored in the body's fatty tissues, or they may be sent to other areas such as the mucous membranes found on the skin, mouth, ears, throat, lungs, intestines, and genitals. These areas are a welcome breeding ground for infectious microbes. The immune system, burdened under toxic load, cannot efficiently fight back. If a virus is present, the virus lodges itself in different areas of the body, penetrating healthy cells and reproducing. The end result is an infection that causes pain, fever, swelling, or other symptoms.

How to prevent infections by building immunity

Infections can best be forestalled by building a strong immune system. To maintain a sound immune system, the body needs exercise and balanced nutrition which includes vitamins, minerals, water, amino acids, antioxidants, essential fatty acids, and enzymes. For the most part, the body is unable to manufacture these elements for itself. We rely on a balanced diet to supply them.

A balanced diet includes liberal amounts of "nature made" fruits and vegetables. Fruits are valued because they are nutritious and add bulk to the diet. They help the body detoxify. Vegetables are also highly valuable because of the important role they play in helping the body to heal.

Most people do not eat a balanced diet. Modern methods of producing, packaging, and distributing foods destroy most beneficial nutrients. This being the case, it is important to increase the intake of raw fruits and vegetables and to use nutritional supplements.

The key to understanding nutrition is to understand the way components work together. In order for chemical reactions to take place, the needed elements have to be present, and conditions have to be right for the body to use what it has been given. If a nutritional supplement is taken in a form that is not readily absorbed by the body, or, if there are impairments that prevent the body from breaking the supplement down and absorbing it into the blood stream, then the body may not be able to use it and taking the supplement is of little value. In addition, even if the supplement is absorbed, it may not be biologically available for use by the body because missing are the other elements that are needed in order for the chemical reaction to take place. This is why whole foods are so important, because their constituents are usually balanced.

A good diet begins with a balanced meal. A balanced meal consists of the following:

- A large green salad, eaten before the main meal
- One serving of protein
- One serving of starch (baked potato, brown rice)
- One green vegetable
- One vegetable of a different color (red, yellow, or white)

The following items are excluded from a good diet because they lower the immune response:

- Sugar
- White flour
- White rice
- Sugared cereals
- Alcohol
- Tobacco

- Caffeine
- Soft drinks

Your health care practitioner can help you determine your specific nutritional program and the need for supplements. It's important to know not only what nutritional supplements to take, but also the quantity—the amount to take, how frequently to take them, and at what times of the day.

It is important to purchase supplements—including minerals, vitamins, and amino acids—that are of the highest quality. Many different companies make supplements, but not all of them may be beneficial for the person you are or for the particular ailment you have. Work closely with a health practitioner that you trust, someone who has the knowledge, the experience, and the training to advise you authoritatively.

Stress and the immune response

In addition to a sound diet, it is also important to learn to manage stress. Anxiety, stress, and other negative emotions can have a negative impact on the immune system. Emotions, such as deep-seated fears, mistrust of others, anger, trauma and stress, can lower the immune response and leave you susceptible to infections.

In modern society, many people live continuously in a state of stress. Chronic disease, an unhappy marriage, or a bad job situation are examples of conditions that cause chronic, long-term stress. General anxiety and tension are the feelings that accompany stress.

Physical changes caused by stress include high blood pressure, increased heart rate, and muscle tension. As digestion slows, cholesterol levels rise to meet an increased need for cortisone. A rise in cholesterol levels suppresses the immune system and inhibits the formation of white blood vessels to fight disease.

When to see a doctor

Plant medicine is the very best option for dealing with infectious illnesses, but self-care is not advisable. You should be prepared to see a medical doctor or a qualified health care practitioner whenever you have an infection. The reason for this is simple. Infections can be very dangerous. For example, an untreated middle ear infection can lead to permanent loss of hearing. A gonococcal infection of the female reproductive tract can lead to infertility. Pneumonia can kill. You cannot always be sure that you have diagnosed your illness correctly, or that there are no complicating factors. Seeing a physician or a qualified health care practitioner is always good advice.

Chapter 5
How To Use Plant Medicines

*"We can never be smug or overconfident about healing.
Anyone can cover up or rearrange symptoms, or dash
around with big doses of herbs used according to the latest
scientific or popular fad, but cure is a mystery which comes
to us from the hidden vortex of God and Mother Nature.
We do not own it; it comes to us as a dispensation from
beyond."* —Matthew Wood

As we learned in Chapter 2, doctors in France have proven that natural plant medicines can be used successfully to treat infectious diseases. The French doctors have used plant medicines against a wide range of infectious illnesses for more than five decades, and have demonstrated these results under clinical conditions. Plants have been proven effective in healing infections, even in chronic cases and in situations where conventional medications have failed.

Properly used, plant medicines are the safest and the most effective means of overcoming an infection. For success in treatment, you will first need to learn how to select the best plants for a particular condition, and after that, how to apply these medicines correctly to the body. Plant medicines may be ingested, inhaled, or put on the skin. Each path of delivery has its own benefits.

Medicinal plants have multiple therapeutic effects. Some are decongestants, useful for clearing the nasal and bronchial passages of excess mucus; others are expectorants, useful for upper respiratory ailments; still others are anti-allergic, and so on. These qualities enable us to use plants against many types of distressing complaints.

How to choose plant medicines

When using natural medicines to relieve symptoms, first determine the *medicinal effects* that are needed to treat the illness. For persons suffering from a toothache or a headache, choose an *analgesic* essential oil or herb to diminish the pain. If a child has a fever, use a *febrifuge* to regulate the fever or a *sudorific* to increase perspiration and sweating and lower body temperature. If there is coughing, an *antitussive* essential oil or herb can relieve this complaint.

Once you determine the medicinal effects that are needed, choosing the appropriate plant remedy becomes a matter of matching the needs of the person with the known medicinal properties of the plant. Different plant remedies can be selected and combined into one. This is known as a *synergistic blend*.

For example, if you have *cystitis*—a bacterial infection of the urinary bladder—a synergistic blend of essential oils can be created using *antiseptic* oils such as Lemon (*Citrus limon*) or Lime (*Citrus aurantifolia*). Antiseptic essential oils have the ability to destroy and prevent the growth of infectious microbes.

Next, you can combine these with an *anti-inflammatory* essential oil, such as German Chamomile (*Matricaria recutica*). If you are experiencing pain, you may also add an analgesic oil such as Black Pepper (*Piper nigrum*) or Clove Bud (*Syzygium aromaticum*). These several essential oils can be combined into one effective, therapeutic, and synergistic essential oil blend.

A similar process can be used to select a blend of herbal tinctures. For example, you could use the following herbs for cystitis:

- Bilberry (*Vaccinium myrtillus*)
- Goldenrod (*Solidago virgaurea*)
- Horsetail (*Equisetum arvense*)

Bilberry is an antiseptic for the urinary tract. It acts against the microorganisms that cause cystitis. It is also a diuretic herb, working specifically on the kidneys and urinary tract to stimulate increased urination. Goldenrod is a gentle astringent herb that can stanch bleeding and has a binding effect on wounds. Horsetail is also an astringent; it is rich in silica and minerals that help repair damaged tissue and reduce inflammation.

When these three herbs are combined, they make a potent formula for someone with cystitis. And when the herbs are also combined with essential oils, the formula is even more powerful. *This is the reason French doctors utilize both essential oils and herbal tinctures simultaneously in treating infections. The medical results obtained with this combined approach are excellent.* Usually up to three essential oils and three different herbal tinctures are selected in a formula designed to meet the specific needs of a patient. However, sometimes single essential oils and herbs are used instead of combination remedies.

Combining herbal tinctures with essential oils

Liquid herbals (herbal tinctures) are usually ingested. When ingested, they work efficiently and fast. Dosages may vary, but taking between 2 and 4 milliliters (2–4 ml.) of an herbal tincture three times per day is typical.

In the U.S., the liquid herbal is normally added to some water or juice, and then swallowed. In France, the practice is somewhat different because essential oils are used along with the herbal tincture.

Two separate formulas are prepared by the French pharmacist. One formula consists of liquid herbals; the other is a diluted blend of essential oils. Although these formulas are not combined in the same bottle, the patient takes both remedies at the same time.

The patient takes these remedies according to the specific dosages prescribed by the doctor—for example, 40 drops of the herbal combination, taken with a half glass of warm water, three times per day. The patient uses a dropper to count how many drops of the liquid herbal to put into the water. The essential oils are used in the same way. A certain number of drops are counted out and added to the same glass of water that holds the herbal tinctures. The patient then swallows the essential oils and herbs together with the water.

Ingesting essential oils

Ingesting essential oils is recommended when the *target organs* (parts of the body you want to reach) are in the gastrointestinal tract (GI tract). These include the mouth, the throat, the stomach, the intestines, and their associated glands and organs. Taking essential oils internally makes sense when you want the oils to interact with the liver and kidneys. Essential oils may be taken orally to fight bladder infections or other infections of the urinary and genital areas.[1]

When essential oils are ingested, they pass through the GI tract and travel to the liver. The liver metabolizes the essential oil molecules, linking them chemically with other molecules and transforming them into a water-soluble state. They are then eliminated from the body.[2]

Most essential oils are safe to use internally as long as the proper instructions are followed. However, aromatherapy literature in America and England cautions about ingesting certain kinds of essential oils. Essential oils high in *phenols* are caustic. When used incorrectly, they can burn and irritate sensitive tissues of the body, including the mucous membranes that line the mouth, the esophagus, and the stomach. Essential oils high in phenols include the antibiotic oils we discussed in Chapter 2: Oregano, Thyme, Cinnamon Bark, and Clove Bud. Besides these, there are other caustic essential oils.

Do not ingest any caustic essential oils without first diluting them. If this is not done, the oil may burn sensitive mucus membranes found in the mouth, esophagus, and stomach. Essential oils can be diluted into honey, a carrier oil such as Sweet Almond, Grapeseed or Olive oil, an alcohol-base herbal tincture, or liquor such as brandy, rum, or vodka.

Honey is often used to give essential oils to children. When honey is used, some people dilute the honey with a little warm water before adding the essential oils. Some recommend raw honey because commercially processed honey may contain undesirable additives.

Carrier oils are generally used for applying essential oils on the skin. However, in certain situations they can also be used internally. Some people prefer carrier oils rather than alcohol, especially when treating children.

When an alcohol-base herbal tincture is used to dilute essential oils, the healing constituents of the herb are combined with the essential oils. This makes the formula more therapeutic and potent. Elderberry, Linden, and Papaya are excellent tinctures to use with essential oils.

Alcoholic drinks are very practical to use for diluting essential oils. The essential oils completely dissolve into the alcohol. When a few drops of the essential oil/alcohol mixture is added to a glass of water, the oils do not float on top of the water as is the case when a carrier oil is used.

When taking essential oils internally, use them with care. In addition to being diluted before ingestion, the treatments should be taken in small doses and only for a limited period of time. If excessive amounts of essential oils are ingested, adverse effects including nausea, vomiting, and fatigue may result.

On the other hand, if usage guidelines are followed, ingestion of therapeutic essential oils is an excellent method of delivering them to the body. English aromatherapists Shirley and Les Price advise limiting the oral use of essential oils for an adult to three drops, three times per day, for no more than three weeks.[3] Other practitioners have similar guidelines.

Using essential oils through inhalation

Another simple and widely used method for administering essential oils is through inhalation. This route provides three ways for the essential oils to gain access to the body:

- Essential oils can be absorbed and enter circulation directly through the blood vessels that line your nose.
- The oils can be inhaled through your nose and eventually reach your lungs where exchange with the blood occurs.
- The constituents of the essential oils are volatile (they evaporate easily) and bind to receptors in the lining of the nose that detect scent, which can then affect your emotions, your mood, and your behavior.

The *olfactory system* controls your sense of smell. Essential oils exert their psychological influence primarily through the olfactory system. When essential oils stimulate the olfactory nerves, impulses travel to the brain. The area of the brain where these signals are received are also the same pathways that affect memory, wakefulness, sleep, emotions, and sexuality.

People can have learned psychological responses to essential oils by associating them with specific experiences. The memory of these experiences evokes the psyche. The sensation of peppermint odor itself can bring back a flood of emotions for almost anyone. What are the smells that remind you of holidays spent at Grandmother's house or of special trips to the beach or mountains? What does the smell of icing on a birthday cake remind you of? Think of the important events in your life. Could your life story be told in smells?

There are several ways to inhale essential oils so that they have a direct effect on the body.

One way to inhale essential oils is to place 2–3 drops of an essential oil on a cloth, tissue, or cotton ball and inhale. This method works well with a fussy baby or an elderly person who may be weak. If the essential oil has sedative qualities (as does Lavender, for example) this method can work quickly, in just a few minutes, to calm and balance the body.

Another way to inhale is to rub 2–4 drops of essential oils into the palms of your hands. Cup your hands over your nose and breathe slowly and deeply. This is extremely effective for relieving sinus and chest congestion. A person experiencing heart palpations can inhale Peppermint essential oil, which performs well in calming an irregular heart beat.

One of the most effective methods of essential oil inhalation is through the use of a cool mist *electric diffusor.* This device breaks apart the already small molecules of the essential oils and disperses them into the air with a gentle force. A good electric diffusor can reach an area of up to 2,000 square feet. Citrus essential oils, such as lemon, grapefruit, and orange are excellent choices for use in the diffusor. They not only refresh stale indoor air, but they also are effective against airborne bacteria. By using a diffusor, you create a warm, friendly atmosphere that will welcome guests into your home, office, or business.

There are various diffusor styles available. You want to find one that has no metal parts in contact with the essential oils. If plastic is used in a diffusor, it must be inert so that the essential oils cannot penetrate the porous material.

Another way to inhale essential oils is by means of *steam distillation.* Steam distillation is an effective, gentle way to unclog pores, stimulate blood circulation, and moisturize and disinfect the skin. To use, mix 3–5 drops of essential oils into a bowl of hot water. Sit comfortably and relax with the bowl in front of you. Breathe deeply while bending over the bowl of water. Your head should be covered with a large towel to keep water vapors from escaping into the room. Keep your eyes closed. When the water cools, you're done. Rinse your face with fresh water.

Essential oils for respiratory problems

Inhalation of essential oils is the most effective way of dealing with infections causing respiratory problems. The most common infectious illnesses of the respiratory system are bronchitis, the common cold, influenza, laryngitis, pneumonia, and tuberculosis. Each of these is discussed in greater detail later on. The respiratory organs include the nose, pharynx, larynx, trachea, bronchi, and lungs. The upper respiratory tract is composed of the nose, pharynx, and larynx. The lower respiratory tract contains the trachea, the bronchial tree, and the lungs.

The *respiratory mucosa* is found along the lining of the respiratory tract. The body produces over 125 ml. of respiratory mucus daily. This mucus forms a blanket that covers the lining of the air distribution tubes. As air enters the body, this lining cleanses, warms, and humidifies the air. It removes dust, insects, pollen, bacteria and other contamination before air reaches the lungs.

However, if there is an excess of mucus and the respiratory passages become clogged and swollen, breathing difficulties will result. The excess mucus also provides a haven for unwanted bacterial growth. Use *anticatarrhal* or *mucolytic* essential oils to reduce the build-up of mucus and to clear the nasal passages; use *expectorant* essential oils to clear excess mucus from the lungs; and use *anti-inflammatory* essential oils to reduce inflammation in the respiratory organs.

Dermal application of essential oils

The *integumentary system* includes the skin, the hair, and the nails. Aromatherapy can be very effective when dealing with infectious illnesses related to the integumentary system. However, the dermal application of essential oils is also helpful for many other types of health problems, including conditions not directly related to the skin.

Essential oils can be effectively used for the treatment of skin infections such as acne and eczema. Insect bites, scratches, and wounds can be treated with essential oils because many essential oils have antibacterial properties. For serious injuries, seek medical attention before using essential oils.

When essential oils are applied to the skin, they pass through the skin and are absorbed into the blood. Blood vessels are located near the surface of the skin. These transport the essential oils and circulate them throughout the body to the places where they are needed. One-third of all the body's blood circulates through the skin at any one time. When essential oils are applied to the skin, their effects are felt in the internal organs and throughout the body.

When thinking about your health, remember one rule: avoid putting anything onto the skin that you wouldn't put in your mouth. The skin will absorb into your bloodstream about 60 percent of whatever you apply to it. Chemicals in cosmetics and personal care products applied to the skin kill the friendly bacteria, leaving you vulnerable to attack by disease-causing germs.

How to use carrier oils

Because essential oils are very concentrated plant medicines, most essential oils should not be applied directly on the skin. When using essential oils on the skin, first blend the essential oils with any unscented, chemical-free lotion or cream, or use a *carrier oil* made from a cold-pressed vegetable oil. Do not use mineral oils (baby oil). Mineral oils do not penetrate the skin, and they also inhibit the action of essential oils.

The most common carrier oils are listed below. Because they are edible oils and generally regarded as safe for internal consumption, these carrier oils may be used orally as well as on the skin. They can carry essential oils into the body, or they can carry essential oils to the skin. This may be why they are called "carrier oils." You may purchase these oils at any health food or grocery store.

- Aloe Vera (*Aloe vera*)
- Hazelnut (*Corylus avellana*)
- Apricot Kernel (*Armeniaca vulgaris*)
- Jojoba (*Simmondisa chinensis*)
- Avocado (*Persea gratissima*)
- Olive (*Olea europaea*)
- Carrot (*Daucus carota*)
- Safflower (*Carthamus tinctorias*)
- Calendula (*Calendula officinalis*)
- Sunflower (*Helianthus annuus*)
- Evening Primrose (*Oenethera biennis*)
- Sweet Almond (*Prunus dulcis*)
- Grape Seed (*Vitis vinifera*)
- Wheat Germ (*Triticum vulgare*)

Some herbal companies sell a natural massage lotion or a special blend of mixing oils for use in aromatherapy. You can also make your own blend of carrier oils.

Prepare these blends ahead of time, before they are needed. If stored properly, their shelf life is about six months to one year. Undiluted essential oils have a much longer shelf life, but when they are mixed with a carrier oil, shelf life is shorter because the carrier oils do not last as long as the essential oils. To deal with this, companies that sell mixing oils commercially usually add Vitamin E to their mixing oil blend. Vitamin E is a natural preservative.

There are many different ways of combining and blending carrier oils. If you are not allergic to wheat, you can add Wheat Germ oil to a carrier oil in order to make your own blend of mixing oils last longer on the shelf. Wheat Germ is an oil rich in Vitamin E. An excellent way to use Wheat Germ oil is to mix one part with nine parts of Sweet Almond oil. Or instead of Sweet Almond oil you can also use Grape Seed oil or Hazelnut oil. You have many different choices.

Most citrus essential oils have a shelf life of approximately two years; other essential oils have an indefinite shelf life as long as they are stored at room temperature away from direct light. Essential oils are sold in tinted bottles to protect them from damage by ultraviolet light. To store your carrier oil, you may obtain an amber-colored or UV-protected container from the health food store.

To apply essential oils to small areas of the skin, place a pearl-size drop of lotion or a teaspoon carrier oil in the palm of your hand, mix in 6–8 drops of essential oils, and apply. The best places to apply essential oils are the pulse points of the wrist, the soles of the feet, the palms of the hands, and on the shoulders and the scalp. If there is pain, apply the essential oils on the area of pain, such as the shoulder, back, temple, or forehead.

Carrier oils are never used in a diffusor because they clog the dispersing mechanism. Only pure, undiluted essential oils are used in a diffusor.

Understanding Dilutions

Essential oils are generally used in low dilutions. They can vary in range from 1% (one drop essential oil combined with one hundred drops carrier oil) to as high as 25% (25 drops of essential oils combined with 100 drops of carrier oil). A typical use of an essential oil for a partial body massage is a 5% dilution for an adult, and 2% for a child.

Diluting essential oils is not an exact science. Various kinds of essential oils have different viscosity (density). People also use pipettes or droppers that have different dropper sizes. To add to the confusion, measurement standards differ from country to country.

If you live in the U.S. or Canada, the equivalency chart found below may help. If you live in another country, please check the website at **www.healthpracticebooks.com** for a link that will give you the equivalency information you need.

U.S. EQUIVALENT ESSENTIAL OIL MEASUREMENTS		
ml = milliliter oz = fluid ounce	tsp = teaspoon TBS = tablespoon	
<u>Drops Essential Oil</u>	<u>Ml</u>	<u>Other</u>
25–30	1 ml	1/4 tsp
125–150	5 ml	1 tsp
375–450	15 ml	1 TBS
750–900	30 ml	1 oz

1% dilution: 1 drop essential oil to 5 ml (1 tsp) of carrier oil
2% dilution: 2–3 drops essential oil to 5 ml (1 tsp) of carrier oil
5% dilution: 6–8 drops essential oil to 5 ml (1 tsp) of carrier oil
10% dilution: 12–15 drops essential oil to 5 ml (1 tsp) of carrier oil
25% dilution: 31–37 drops essential oil to 5 ml (1 tsp) of carrier oil

If measuring essential oils by metric weight,
one gram is usually equivalent to one milliliter.

Neat application of essential oils

Certain essential oils are generally not diluted in a carrier oil when applied to small areas of the body. Prominent examples are Lavender and Tea Tree. These essential oils are applied *neat*—or directly, as is—to boils, pimples, warts, or other areas of the skin requiring care.

In addition to Lavender or Tea Tree, there are other essential oils that some people apply neat. Neat application of essential oils is sometimes needed in order to resolve a health problem. In our family, we use essential oils such as Bergamot, Frankincense, Helichrysum, or Lemon without diluting them. We can do this because we do not have a skin sensitivity to these oils, and because we are experienced and understand the action of the oils.

Do not use "hot oils" such as Cinnamon Bark, Clove Bud, Peppermint, Oregano or Thyme neat on your skin, or in aromatherapy baths. Check the usage instructions found in the Appendix for guidance.

It is best to test an essential oil before using it undiluted, especially if you have a light complexion and sensitive skin. Apply one drop of the oil you are testing to your skin (for example, on your wrist at the pulse point) and wait 15 minutes. If an adverse reaction develops, do not use the oil undiluted, or do not use the oil at all.

Never put essential oils directly into the eyes, ears, or other sensitive areas of the body. If you happen to do so, immediately flush the area with milk or a pure vegetable oil. Do not use water, since essential oils are not soluble in water. Water will push the essential oil deeper into the tissue.

How to make a compress

A compress made with essential oils or herbs may be used for muscular aches and pains, arthritis, rheumatism, and menstrual cramps. Cold compresses are effective in the treatment of migraine headaches, for fevers, and to reduce swelling and inflammation of the joints. Hot compresses are used to treat chronic back and muscle pain, spasms, colic, ear aches, and menstrual pain. Alternating hot and cold compresses are used for sprains.

To make a cold compress, use ice-cold water. For a hot compress, do not use boiling water, but use water that is very hot. To make either a hot or cold compress, add 6–8 drops of essential oils or 10–20 drops of an herbal tincture to 3/4 cup of water and agitate to disperse them. Lay a small towel or a flannel cloth over the water to soak up the oils and herbs. Lightly squeeze out any excess water, and apply the towel to the area of pain. You may wrap plastic around the compress and use a small dry towel to cover. Leave the compress until you need to replace it. Some people change the compress every 15 minutes; others leave it on for up to two hours. Do what suits you best.

Massage with essential oils

Massage is one of the most natural and instinctive means of relieving pain and discomfort during illness. When a person has sore muscles, abdominal pains, or a bruise or a wound, the first impulse is to rub or touch the area to obtain relief. Massage stimulates the reflexes, causes muscles to relax, stretches connective tissue, and promotes the circulation of blood and lymph fluids through the tissues.

When massage is combined with aromatherapy, the healing effects of both are enhanced. In addition to its beneficial effects on the body's muscles and ligaments, aromatherapy massage stimulates the body's chemistry and can have positive impact on the emotions.

Aromatherapy massage is one of the best-known measures for dealing with stress. Aromatherapy massage can also relieve anxiety, asthma and insomnia, and is an excellent supportive therapy for people undergoing treatment for addictions.

There are many different types of massage that can be used in conjunction with aromatherapy:

- Acupressure
- Cranio-sacral therapy
- Reflexology
- Shiatsu
- Swedish massage

When using aromatherapy in a full-body massage, first choose a carrier oil or unscented massage lotion. Then mix in the essential oils at a 2% dilution (15–18 drops of essential oils to one fluid ounce of carrier oil). This mixture may be applied to the shoulders, the back, or other large areas of the body.

The aromatherapy bath

One of the easiest ways to use essential oils at home is in the aromatherapy bath or shower. Aromatherapy baths combine the benefits of inhalation with the powers of absorption through the skin. Bathing with essential oils cleans the body and balances the emotions. It can eliminate stress or anxiety, or prepare you for a good night's rest. Bathing is helpful for sore, tight muscles, and tension in the back. It opens clogged sinuses, and can relieve a tension headache.

When adding essential oils to the bath, first dilute the essential oils in a pure bath gel that is free of harmful ingredients. Essential oils are not water soluble and will not fully disperse when added directly to bath water. Instead, the essential oils will float on top of the water unless they are properly diluted.

To use essential oils in a bath, mix 6–8 drops of essential oils to a teaspoon of liquid soap or another base product, then add to running water to disperse. Close the doors and windows so that the vapors from the essential oils remain in the room.

A footbath is another way of bathing with essential oils. A footbath can relax tired and swollen feet, ease the pain of a blister, or treat fungal infections, boils, and ingrown toenails. To use, simply dilute 6–8 drops of essential oils to a teaspoon of base product and add to warm water. Alternatively, you can add the essential oils to a bath gel, apply the gel directly to the feet, and massage. Then soak and relax in warm water for ten minutes.

Guidelines for safety

Most essential oils and herbal medicines are safer to use than drugs. There have been reports about the unsafe use of herbs, but in actuality there have been few illnesses or fatalities where plant medicines were employed.

Some poisonings have occurred as a result of ingesting plants. To the extent that I am aware, these plants were poisonous mushrooms or household plants, not medicinal herbs. The essential oils and herbs listed in this book are not dangerous. However, anything can be risky if used in excess or used incorrectly. Whenever plant medicines are used to treat a problem, always check for any applicable safety information.

It is not necessary to be a doctor to use plant medicines, but plant medicines are always best used under a practitioner's supervision. Practitioners have been trained in the differential diagnosis of illnesses, and they can advise about allergies, drug-herb interactions, and other safety issues.

Most plant medicines are safe to use unless you fall into the categories listed below. These people can still use plant medicines, but they must be especially careful to check the usage charts in the Appendix and avoid using the plant medicines that are contraindicated for their condition:

- Pregnant women or nursing mothers
- People with high blood pressure
- People with allergies to certain types of plants, such as ragweed, milkweed, daisies, etc.
- Diabetics and people with blood sugar problems
- Infants, young children and the elderly
- People who are taking over-the-counter drugs, prescription drugs, or other medications. Be especially cautious about interactions with aspirin or other blood thinning drugs, anticoagulant drugs, and high blood pressure medications
- Epileptic patients

Adjust your dosages according to your age and body weight. If you are not an adult, reduce the dosage. As a general rule, for an adolescent between the ages of 12 and 17, use three-fourths of the recommended amount for an adult. For a child between six and 12, use one-half of the amount. For a child younger than six, use one-fourth of the recommended amount.[4]

It is usually best not administer essential oils to babies under the age of three months. Keep the bottles containing essential oils tightly sealed, out of the reach of children.

Pregnant women should avoid all essential oils during the first trimester. Avoid using Basil, Clary Sage, and Fennel essential oils during any trimester. Lavender and Roman Chamomile essential oils may be used sparingly during the second and third trimesters.

Do not go directly into the sun after applying citrus essential oils to the skin. Ultraviolet rays react with some of the constituents found in citrus essential oils. You could experience inflammation of the skin, or burning. Essential oils that are *photo toxic* include Bergamot, Neroli, Orange, Lime, and Lemon. Unlike other citrus oils, Grapefruit oil is not photo toxic.

You will find a complete list of essential oils and herbs, their common and botanical names, their medicinal usages, and their responsible cautions in the Appendix. Before using any of the formulas described in this book, you should check the there. It is important to understand the safety instructions found in this book before using any essential oils and herbs. Do not use essential oils and herbs if they are contraindicated for your condition.

Essential oils are very concentrated plant medicines; use them according to correct and safe instructions. If you have questions or concerns check with your health care professional.

Chapter 6
When Infections Strike

*"It is conceivable that the day will come when the true
therapeutic value of natural substances will be given proper
recognition.... Future generations will doubtlessly be as
nonplussed by certain theories and medical teachings that
today occupy a respectable position as we are by the
treatment for scabies common in the 18th century."*
—Jean Valnet

In this chapter will be found an alphabetical list of common infectious illnesses. They include bacterial, viral, and fungal infections, as well as infections caused by parasites and worms. Under each illness will first be found a brief description of characteristic causes and symptoms. Next, there will be lists of the most effective essential oils and herbal tinctures to use, followed by safety information and instructions for treatment. In addition, there are recommendations for adjusting the diet, for detoxifying the body, and other measures that may prove helpful.

To begin using herbal medicines, it is first necessary to obtain a few supplies:

1. Essential oils
2. Herbal tinctures
3. One or more carrier oils to dilute the essential oils
4. A tinted glass container to store your carrier oil
5. A few empty 2-ounce tinted glass bottles equipped with a dropper.
6. A cool mist, electric diffusor
7. Vegetable capsules (gel caps)
8. Raw Lavender honey (optional)
9. Vodka, Rum, or Brandy (this is also optional)
10. Cotton swabs

Vegetable capsules, glass container, honey and empty 2-ounce dropper bottles can be purchased at the health food store. For the remaining supplies, locate a reliable source. (Visit the internet site at **www.healthpracticebooks.com** for suggestions on where to obtain medicinal quality essential oils and herbs.)

Obtain the necessary supplies in order to begin using essential oils and herbs properly. In the instructions that follow, examples of synergistic herbal blends and various options for using essential oils with specific types of infectious illnesses are given.

For some of the illnesses that are listed, the instructions call for taking liquid herbals internally while using essential oils externally, through inhalation or dermal application. Illnesses associated with the respiratory system are handled in this way, as well as disorders of the integumentary system (the skin, hair, and nails).

For most other illnesses, the instructions require taking essential oils internally along with ingesting the liquid herbals. To do this properly, first dilute the essential oils as instructed. Honey, honey water, a carrier oil, an herbal tincture, or an alcoholic drink such as vodka or brandy can be used as the dilution medium. This mixture can be added to the liquid herbal in water after the essential oils have been diluted in the proper proportion.

Herbal medicines are being used in their optimum way when herbal tinctures and essential oils are taken together in the treatment of a particular condition. Essential oils and herbal tinctures may be used internally or externally in any number of different ways, but using both types of plant medicine at the same time will yield a noticeable difference in results.

To avoid needless repetition, the following abbreviations are used in the text:

HT   Herbal Tincture
EO   Essential Oil
ΔΔ   Safety information or use caution. These are listed in the footnotes, and also in Appendix A and B.

ABSCESSES

An abscess is a localized build-up of pus caused by infection. Abscesses may be located internally or externally, and can be found in any tissue of the body. When they are near the surface of the skin, they are characterized by pain, tenderness, and a mass with a red, firm surface and a soft center.

An abscess about the root of a tooth is usually the result of an infection of dental pulp following dental caries. Abscesses developing in the liver occur as a complication of amebic dysentery. Abscesses may also form in the brain, lungs, abdominal wall, gastrointestinal tract, ears, tonsils, sinuses, breasts, kidneys, prostate gland, mouth, and gums.

Abscesses result from infection by bacteria, viruses, parasites, or fungi. They may be accompanied by fatigue, loss of appetite, weight loss, and alternating episodes of fever and chills. If symptoms are severe they may indicate septicemia, the presence of bacteria in the blood. If abscesses are slow to appear and symptoms are mild, this may signal a chronic condition.

Do not wait for the abscess to burst or drain. Begin treatment immediately as soon as it appears.

INSTRUCTIONS FOR EXTERNAL APPLICATION
Lavender (*Lavandula angustifolia*) *EO*

- Rub one drop of Lavender directly on the infected area. Do not spread the oil over a large area of skin; dab directly on the abscess with a cotton swab. Do not rub in vigorously. Repeat three to five times per day. Discontinue treatment if rash or irritation appears.
- Lavender may be used in a compress.
- If the abscess is severe, cover the affected area with gauze bandage that has been soaked in essential oils. Leave on for 6–8 hours. Continue until healing is complete.[1]

DIRECTIONS FOR INTERNAL USE
Burdock (*Arctium lappa*) *HT* ΔΔ

- Use according to label instructions or add 10–30 drops to a half-glass of water or juice. Take 10 minutes before meals, three times per day.

Other useful essential oils: *Basil, Bergamot, German Chamomile, Lemon, Pine Needle, Tea Tree.*
Suggestions: *see Fevers (p. 127), Mouth Infections (p. 155).*

ΔΔ Burdock HT: If taking insulin or medications to lower blood sugar, Burdock may increase their effects. Use Slippery Elm (*Ulmus rubra*) HT instead.

ACNE

Acne occurs most frequently during adolescence. Between the ages of 10 and 19, the sebaceous glands increase their secretion. The gland ducts become blocked by oil and dead skin cells, causing inflammation and attracting bacteria. Acne can affect people of all ages, men as well as women. In women, acne outbreaks are common during the onset of the menstrual cycle.

The most common infectious agents causing acne are staph, strep, and *Candida albicans*. White blood cells fight off infections, causing inflammation or swelling. Pimples form on the face, back, and shoulders. Constant skin eruptions can cause scars.

Stress, poor diet, hormonal imbalances and food allergies can also cause acne. When the liver and kidneys are overloaded and no longer eliminate sufficiently, the body eliminates toxins through the skin.

INSTRUCTIONS FOR EXTERNAL APPLICATION
Bergamot (*Citrus bergamia*) EO ΔΔ
Cedarwood Atlas (*Cedrus atlantica*) EO ΔΔ
Lavender (*Lavandula augustifolia*) EO
Tea Tree (*Melaleuca alternifolia*) EO

- Select one to three essential oils to use. Wash the face and affected areas at least two times per day with 6–8 drops of one or more of the above essential oils mixed with a teaspoon liquid soap. After cleaning, dab a single drop of essential oil directly to the pustule or lesion caused by acne. Do not spread essential oil over a large area of the skin; do not rub in vigorously. Discontinue use if the skin becomes irritated.

• Use a facial sauna to unblock pores and clear the skin: mix 3–5 drops of any of above essential oils into a bowl of hot water. Sit and relax with the bowl in front of you. Breathe deeply while bending over the bowl of water. Keep your head covered with a large towel to keep the water vapors from escaping into the room. When finished, rinse face with fresh water.[2]

• To reduce scarring as a result of acne, apply Lavender neat to the affected area on a daily basis until the scar diminishes.

DIRECTIONS FOR INTERNAL USE
Burdock *(Arctium lappa)* HT ∆∆
Dandelion *(Taraxacum dens leonis or T. officinale)* HT ∆∆
Yellow Dock *(Rumex crispus)* HT ∆∆

• Select one to three herbal tinctures. Use according to label instructions or add 10 to 30 drops to a half-glass of water or juice. If taking two herbal tinctures, add 10 to 15 drops of each, and if taking three herbal tinctures, add 10 drops of each. Take 10 minutes before meals, three times per day.

Other useful essential oils: *Geranium, Lemon, Pine Needle*
Other useful herbal tinctures: *Echinacea, Oregon Grape, Red Clover, Slippery Elm.*
Suggestions: *Do not pick at the skin or squeeze pustules and pimples. Avoid foods that, according to your experience, cause acne to worsen. Periodic fasting may be helpful. Eat vegetables. Do not use greasy ointments on your skin. Regular exercise stimulates circulation to the skin and improves the immune response. Deficiencies of Vitamin B have been linked to acne, so supplementing with a good quality B multi-vitamin supplement may be helpful.*

∆∆ Bergamot EO: do not go into direct sunlight after applying to the skin.
∆∆ Burdock HT: may enhance the effect of insulin or blood sugar lowering medications.

ΔΔ Cedarwood Atlas EO: do not use if pregnant.

ΔΔ Dandelion HT: do not use without doctor's permission if you have stomach ulcers or gastritis.

ΔΔ Yellow Dock HT: contraindicated for pregnancy, may cause diarrhea or nausea.

ANTHRAX

Anthrax is an acute infectious disease caused by the naturally occurring *Bacillus anthracis*, a bacteria that is found in soil. Anthrax normally affects sheep, cattle, and other livestock. People can contract anthrax from contact with animal hair, hides, or waste. The usual, accidental way of human exposure to anthrax is through the skin. As a weapon of biological warfare, anthrax spores are spread through inhalation or direct physical contact. A lethal dose of anthrax is only one-millionth of a gram. An aerosol cloud of lethal anthrax spores would be colorless, odorless and invisible, and would affect people indoors as well as outdoors.

Skin anthrax, the most common form, resembles a reddish pimple or bug bite at the onset. After a day or two, it becomes a fluid-filled sac. Over the next seven to ten days it forms an ulcerous scab with a black center. The surrounding skin swells, looking gangrenous. There will be burning pain. Eventually, the ulcer will discharge a foul-smelling pus. The patient will have intense thirst and fever.

Respiratory anthrax at first resembles the flu. The first stage, which lasts from anywhere from a few hours to a few days, consists of fatigue, fever and chills, thirst, vomiting, diarrhea, and pain in the abdomen and chest. This is followed by a brief period of recovery.

The second stage of respiratory anthrax is violent, with sudden fever, difficult breathing, intense sweating, delirium, hemorrhaging from the lungs and massive swelling. The skin will turn blue.

Eighty percent of anthrax victims die within days. For treatment to be effective, antibiotic medicines must be taken within 48 hours of exposure. However, some types of anthrax are resistant to antibiotics. Essential oils and herbs are traditional ways of treating anthrax. Use both essential oils and herbal tinctures as quickly as possible after onset of symptoms to increase the chances of survival.

INSTRUCTIONS FOR EXTERNAL APPLICATION (FOR SKIN ANTHRAX)

- To use essential oils externally on skin ulcers, use the same essential oils that are listed to treat Abscesses. Apply these directly on the ulcers as instructed.

DIRECTIONS FOR INTERNAL USE (FOR SKIN ANTHRAX)

Cinnamon Bark *(Cinnamomum zeylanicum)* EO ∆∆
Lavender *(Lavandula augustifolia)* EO
Geranium *(Pelargonium graveolens)* EO
Savory *(Satureja hortensis)* EO ∆∆

- Add 5 drops Cinnamon Bark, 8 drops Geranium, 5 drops Lavender, and 5 drops Savory to 2 ounce bottle of vodka or brandy. Add 40–50 drops of this EO/alcohol mixture to a half-glass of warm water. Then add 20 drops of each of the following herbs into the water:

Calendula *(Calendula officinalis)* HT
Artichoke *(Cynara scolymus)* HT ∆∆

- Take combined mixture three times per day, before meals.

INSTRUCTIONS FOR EXTERNAL APPLICATION (FOR RESPIRATORY ANTHRAX)

- See Bronchitis, p. 102.

DIRECTIONS FOR INTERNAL USE (FOR RESPIRATORY ANTHRAX)

Lavender *(Lavandula augustifolia)* EO
Oregano *(Oreganum vulgare)* EO

- Add 45 drops of each of the above essential oils to a 2 ounce bottle vodka or brandy. Add 40–50 drops of this EO/alcohol mixture to a half-glass of warm water. Then add 10 to 12 drops of each of the following herbs to the water:

Echinacea *(Echinacea angustifolia or E. purpurea)* HT ΔΔ
Elderberry *(Sambucus nigra)* HT
Garlic *(Allium sativum)* HT ΔΔ
Goldenseal *(Hydrastis canadensis)* HT ΔΔ

- Take combined mixture three times per day, 10 minutes before meals.

FOR USE IN THE DIFFUSOR TO DISINFECT THE HOUSE/ROOM AIR
Clove Bud *(Syzygium aromaticum)* EO
Lemon *(Citrus limon)* or Lime *(Citrus aurantifolia)* EO ΔΔ

- Add 20 drops Clove Bud to a 15 ml. bottle Lemon *(Citrus limon)* or Lime *(Citrus aurantifolia)* and use in an electric diffusor.

Suggestions: *Isolate the patient and give complete bed rest. Contact health authorities and follow stringent disinfection procedures. All bed linens, towels, and clothing should be sterilized, and the room should be disinfected.*

ΔΔ Artichoke HT: contraindicated for pregnancy, kidney and liver disease.
ΔΔ Cinnamon Bark EO: avoid during pregnancy, do not apply to the skin undiluted.
ΔΔ Echinacea HT: avoid if allergic to ragweed.
ΔΔ Garlic HT: thins the blood. Do not use if on anti-coagulant drugs.
ΔΔ Goldenseal HT: do not use excessively (more than 3 times daily) or long term (more than 7 days). Contraindicated for pregnancy, hypertension, low blood sugar, allergy to ragweed.
ΔΔ Lemon EO: do not go into direct sunlight after using on skin.
ΔΔ Oregano EO: do not use if pregnant.
ΔΔ Savory EO: do not use if pregnant.

ATHLETE'S FOOT, NAIL FUNGUS, RINGWORM

Ringworm is a common term for a fungal skin infection. "Athlete's foot," or "ringworm of the feet" are common but misleading names for *Tinea pedis*, a fungal infection of the dead skin on the surface of the feet. A worm does not cause this condition. Anyone can be susceptible, not just athletes. When people's feet come in contact with warm, moist surfaces, the infection spreads readily. Other forms of ringworm are found on the scalp (*Tinea capitis*), the body (*Tinea corporis*), the beard (*Tinea barbae*), and the nails (*Tinea unguium*).

Ringworm is caused by the dermatophyte fungus, which invades the skin directly or enters through cuts and cracks. The fungus feeds on keratin, a protein found in the skin, hair, and nails. It also feeds on glucose, a form of sugar found in the blood. Athlete's foot usually begins in the webbing between the fourth and fifth toes. It then spreads to other areas. Inflammation, blisters, cracking skin, itching and scaling are the characteristic symptoms.

Dermatophyte is difficult to eradicate because the fungus has special defenses against the body's immune response. Without treatment, the body usually cannot rid itself of this fungus. An "inside out" approach is needed. The "inside" part of the treatment makes the body an inhospitable place for the fungus to grow. The "outside" part attacks and kills the fungus directly.

The recommendations below can be effective against ringworm, but be aware that progress takes time. The treatment can last weeks. Be persistent while anticipating gradual improvements.

INSTRUCTIONS FOR EXTERNAL APPLICATION
Lavender (*Lavandula augustifolia*) *EO*
Tea Tree (*Melaleuca alternifolia*) *EO*

- Use the above essential oils undiluted. For athlete's foot and ringworm on the scalp or the body, spot treat by applying 6–8 drops essential oils to affected area two or three times per day. Be liberal in the amounts used and continue daily treatments until the condition clears. This may take several weeks. Combine with herbal tinctures taken internally.
- To prevent transmitting foot fungus to groin area, put socks on before putting on underwear when dressing. If you already have fungal infection in the groin area, treat both areas simultaneously.

Oregano *(Oreganum vulgare)* ΔΔ

- To treat athlete's foot or nail fungus, prepare a mixture consisting of one part Oregano essential oil to three parts carrier oil. Apply liberally to the affected areas daily. For nail fungus, apply over and under the infected nail. Continue using for a month or longer until the area of new nail growth reaches the area of infection.

DIRECTIONS FOR INTERNAL USE
Astragalus *(Astragalus membranaceus)* HT
Echinacea *(Echinacea angustifolia or E. purpurea)* HT ΔΔ
Goldenseal *(Hydrastis canadensis)* ΔΔ

- Select one to three herbal tinctures. Use according to label instructions or add 10 to 30 drops to a half glass of water or juice. Take 10 minutes before meals, three times per day.

Suggestions: *Adjust the diet. See Candida Albicans (p. 108) for more information.*

ΔΔ Echinacea HT: avoid if allergic to ragweed.
ΔΔ Goldenseal HT: do not use excessively (more than 3 times daily) or long term (longer than 7 days) contraindicated for pregnancy, hypertension, low blood sugar, allergy to ragweed.
ΔΔ Oregano EO: do not use if pregnant. Do not use in the area of the groin; instead, use Lavender EO or Tea Tree EO.

BITES AND STINGS

In 1903, British army surgeon Sir Ronald Ross proved that malaria was transmitted to man via the female Anopheles mosquito. Since that time, numerous other infectious illnesses have been associated with insect bites and stings. To name just a few, the tsetse fly transmits African sleeping sickness, fleas carried by rats transmit plague, and the common house fly can be a carrier of typhoid fever.

Most bites by mosquitoes, fleas, or gnats are relatively harmless. However, ticks can spread Rocky Mountain spotted fever and Lyme disease (see Lyme Disease, p. 150).

Insects that sting include ants, bees, hornets, yellow jackets, wasps, and spiders. More people die each year from insect bites than from the bite of any other poisonous animal.

When an insect stings, it injects venom through its stinger into the victim. The sting causes swelling, redness, pain, and burning in the area of contact. Most stings are harmless, but some people are allergic and can have a severe reaction. Symptoms include hoarseness, difficulty swallowing, labored breathing, weakness, shock, and the closing of an airway.

Insects sting humans when threatened or attacked. Multiple stings suffered from swarms of bees, wasps, or yellow jackets can create a medical emergency. Take care not to interfere with the activity of a hive, unless you are properly prepared with protective clothing and equipment. Also do not squash a dead yellow jacket; their bodies release a chemical that calls other yellow jackets to the attack.

If a stinger is left in the skin, it must be removed to stop the swelling. Do not attempt to lift the stinger out with your fingers or a tweezer. This could cause you to inadvertently release more venom into the body from the venom sac attached to the stinger. Instead, using a sterilized knife or a similar object, carefully scrape the stinger out.

In the case of an insect sting, take the patient to the doctor and treat it as a medical emergency if any of the following symptoms appear: severe pain, sudden and severe swelling of the lips, tongue, eyes, or body, itching all over the body, hives, wheezing, coughing, trouble breathing, dizziness and weakness, nausea and vomiting, and collapse.

In the U.S., there are two types of spiders that cause harm to humans. The black widow spider has a black body and a red hourglass shape on the main body. The recluse spider creates a "bull's eye" blister, consisting of red and white rings that encircle each other. The bite of a black widow spider is painful and sharp. They often infest outhouses and bite their victims in the buttocks or genitals.

Bites by poisonous spiders constitute a medical emergency requiring immediate treatment. If no medical care is available, administer first aid as explained in the following instructions.

Similarly, bites by scorpions require immediate medical care. Scorpions have elongated bodies and curly tails.

Dog bites that break the skin are dangerous because of the risk of rabies or tetanus infection. Find out if the dog has been immunized against rabies. If no records are available, alert health authorities and keep the dog under observation for signs of viciousness, foaming at the mouth, agitation, or paralysis. If the dog cannot be found or if no record of immunization is available, the human victim will require injections to prevent rabies. Get a tetanus injection.

There are approximately two dozen species poisonous snakes in the U.S. Some species are only mildly toxic; others create paralysis, unconsciousness, and death. Typical symptoms include swelling, discoloration of the skin in the area of the bite, weakness, racing pulse, shortness of breath, nausea, and vomiting.

The bite by a poisonous snake is a medical emergency. Seek immediate medical care, even if the initial symptoms do not appear serious. If medical care is not available, administer first aid (see below). Snake bites are more serious in the case of young children and the elderly.

INSTRUCTIONS FOR EXTERNAL APPLICATION

Lavender (*Lavandula augustifolia*) EO
Tea Tree (*Melaleuca alternifolia*) EO

- Spot treat area of bite or sting. You may also make a compress with these essential oils.
- If you have been bitten by a dog, wash the area thoroughly with warm water and 6–8 drops essential oils mixed with a teaspoon of liquid soap. If necessary, cover affected area with gauze bandage that has been soaked in essential oils for 24 hours.
- For snake and poisonous spider bites, seek immediate medical help. In the meantime, keep the patient as calm as possible. Apply liberal amounts of Lavender to the wound. Immobilize the area of the bite by applying a constricting band two to four inches above the bite. If possible, keep the injured area below heart level. In an extreme situation, if there is rapid swelling and medical help is not available or delayed, make an incision directly below the fang marks. Use a sharp, sterilized blade. Cut just through the skin, about one-eighth inch deep, a half-inch long. Apply suction for at least 30 minutes using a suction cup, or suck with the mouth,

spitting out the blood. In life or death situations, massive doses of Vitamin C may be helpful. Do not apply ice packs to avoid damaging tissue. For follow-up care, see Wound Healing, p. 181.

TO MAKE AN INSECT REPELLANT

Citronella *(Cymbopogon nardus) EO* ΔΔ
Cedarwood Atlas *(Cedrus atlantica) EO* ΔΔ
Eucalyptus *(Eucalyptus globulus) EO*
Geranium *(Pelargonium graveolens) EO*
Lavender *(Lavandula augustifolia) EO*
Lemongrass *(Cymbopogon citratus) EO* ΔΔ

• Add 10 drops of each of the above essential oils to 1/4 cup water mixed with a liquid emulsifier (for example, hair conditioner). Place mixture into a spray bottle. Shake before each use and spray. Apply to face, neck, ears, arms, or legs, or on clothes. Safe for children and pets.

INSTRUCTIONS FOR EXTERNAL APPLICATION

Comfrey *(Symphytum officinale) HT* ΔΔ
Slippery Elm *(Ulmus fulva) HT*
Plantain *(Plantago major) HT*

• Select one to three herbal tinctures. Make a cold compress and apply to area of injury.

DIRECTIONS FOR INTERNAL USE TO BOOST IMMUNE FUNCTION

Cat's Claw *(Uncaria tomentosa) HT* ΔΔ
Echinacea *(Echinacea angustifolia or E. purpurea) HT* ΔΔ
Garlic *(Allium sativum) HT* ΔΔ

• Select one to three of the above tinctures. Use according to label instructions or add 10 to 30 drops to a half-glass of water or juice. If taking two herbal tinctures, add 10 to 15 drops of each, and if taking three herbal tinctures, add 10 drops of each. Take 10 minutes before meals, three times per day.

ΔΔ Cat's Claw HT: contraindicated for pregnancy, hemophiliacs, organ transplant patients.

ΔΔ Cedarwood Atlas EO: contraindicated for pregnancy.

ΔΔ Citronella EO: contraindicated for pregnancy, skin irritant.

ΔΔ Comfrey HT: not to be taken internally without doctor's permission.

ΔΔ Echinacea HT: avoid if allergic to ragweed.

ΔΔ Garlic HT: thins the blood. Do not use if on anti-coagulant drugs.

ΔΔ Lemongrass EO: may irritate the skin in some people.

BOILS

Boils or furuncles are usually a bacterial infection of the hair follicles characterized by inflamed pustules. A simple furuncle has a single core and may be no more than a pimple. When these fuse into a mass of boils or even larger areas of pus-filled lesions, they are called carbuncles. They arise from within the deepest layer of the skin, the subcutaneous layer. The deep-tissue inflammation can be so severe that blood clots form. This causes the formation of a dead, pus-filled core that the body eventually wants to either expel or reabsorb.

Boils are very common among children and adolescents. People with diabetes or kidney disease may be especially susceptible to repeated attacks. Boils appear where hair roots are chafed or irritated, usually on the scalp, buttocks, face, or under the arms. They can be very painful. They may appear suddenly, appearing first as an inflammation that is tender and painful. There may be itching and localized swelling. Within 24 hours, the boil becomes red and filled with pus. Nearby lymph glands may swell.

Boils are very contagious. When the pus drains from an open boil, it can contaminate nearby skin causing new boils to appear. The infection can also enter the bloodstream and infect other parts of the body. Without treatment, a boil usually comes to a head, opens, drains and heals in 10 to 25 days. With treatment, symptoms are less severe and new boils do not appear.

INSTRUCTIONS FOR EXTERNAL APPLICATION
Bergamot *(Citrus bergamia)* EO ΔΔ
Hyssop *(Hyssopus officinalis)* EO ΔΔ
Tea Tree *(Melaleuca alternifolia)* EO

• Do not wait for the boil to burst. Apply essential oils directly on the infected area as soon as problem appears. Mix essential oils with a carrier oil using a 5% dilution. (To calculate dilutions, see page 82.) Do not spread essential oils over a large area of skin; just dab on the boil with a cotton swab. Do not rub in vigorously. Discontinue treatment if rash or irritation appears.

• If the boil is severe, cover affected area with gauze bandage that has been soaked in essential oils, leave on for 6–8 hours. Continue this treatment until healing is complete.[3]

DIRECTIONS FOR INTERNAL USE
Echinacea *(Echinacea angustifolia or E. purpurea)* HT ∆∆
Elderberry *(Sambucus nigra)* HT
Garlic *(Allium sativum)* HT ∆∆
Goldenseal *(Hydrastis canadensis)* HT ∆∆

• Select one to four herbal tinctures. Use according to label instructions or add 10 to 30 drops to a half glass of water or juice. Take 10 minutes before meals, three times per day.

Other useful essential oils: *Lemon, Niaouli, Thyme.*
Other useful herbal tinctures: *Astragalus, Black Walnut, Burdock.*
Suggestions: *Boils should not be pinched or squeezed, especially if they appear on the face or on the ear. Pinching can cause the infection to spread. If boils are large or persistent, see a doctor.*

∆∆ Bergamot EO: do not go into direct sunlight after using on skin.
∆∆ Echinacea HT: avoid if allergic to ragweed.
∆∆ Garlic HT: thins blood. Consult doctor if on anticoagulant drugs.
∆∆ Hyssop HT: contraindicated for pregnancy and epilepsy.
∆∆ Goldenseal HT: do not use excessively (more than 3 times daily) or long term (longer than 7 days); contraindicated for pregnancy, hypertension, low blood sugar, allergy to ragweed.

BRONCHITIS

Bronchitis is an inflammation of the mucous membranes of the bronchi (lung airways), resulting in a persistent cough that produces large quantities of phlegm.

Acute bronchitis is a temporary condition caused by infection. It is often preceded by the common cold or an upper respiratory tract infection, such as influenza. Symptoms include chest and back pain, fatigue, sore throat, chills, and shaking. Most cases of acute bronchitis heal themselves within two weeks, but the condition can also progress, leading to pneumonia. This is most likely to occur if the patient is already weak from a chronic respiratory disease or some other debilitating illness.

Chronic bronchitis is a long-lasting condition characterized by swelling of the respiratory tract and excessive mucus production, which blocks air passages. People with chronic bronchitis have difficulty with exhaling and often cough deeply as they try to dislodge the accumulating mucus.

The major cause of chronic bronchitis is cigarette smoking or exposure to cigarette smoke. Exposure to other air pollutants may also cause chronic bronchitis. Chronic bronchitis is dangerous because as lung function decreases, the heart must compensate in order to maintain the body's homeostasis. Over time, this can lead to hypertension, enlargement of the heart, and heart failure.

INSTRUCTIONS FOR EXTERNAL APPLICATION
For topical use, aromatherapy bath, diffusor or steam inhalation:
Bergamot *(Citrus bergamia)* EO ΔΔ
Eucalyptus *(Eucalyptus globulus)* EO
Tea Tree *(Melaleuca alternifolia)* EO

- Partial body massage: select one to three of the above essential oils. Apply to the chest, back, and the bottoms of the feet. Use 2% dilution for infants and young children. For teens and adults, use a 5% dilution or apply neat if this does not irritate the skin. To calculate dilutions, see page 82.

INSTRUCTIONS FOR EXTERNAL APPLICATION
For a 3-month-old or older baby:[4]
Cypress *(Cupressus sempervirens)* EO
Lavender *(Lavandula augustifolia)* EO
Tea Tree *(Melaleuca alternifolia)* EO

- Mix 10–12 drops of each of the previous essential oils into a 2-ounce bottle Sweet Almond carrier oil. Use topically as a partial body massage.

DIRECTIONS FOR INTERNAL USE[5]
Lavender *(Lavandula augustifolia)* EO
Tea Tree *(Melaleuca alternifolia)* EO
Thyme *(Thymus serpyllum)* EO ΔΔ
Wild Rosemary *(Rosmariunus officinalis)* EO ΔΔ

- Combine 7–8 drops Lavender, 7–8 drops Tea Tree, 12–13 drops Thyme, and 12–13 drops Wild Rosemary with a 2-ounce bottle vodka or brandy. Take 30–40 drops of this mixture with herbal tinctures (see below) in water, three times per day before each meal.

For an adult with acute bronchitis:
Black Currant *(Ribes nigrum)* HT
Wild Cherry Bark *(Prunus Serotina)* HT

For a baby with acute bronchitis:
Black Currant *(Ribes nigrum)* HT
Horsetail *(Equisetum arvense)* HT ΔΔ

For a young child with acute bronchitis:
Angelica *(Angelica archangelica)* HT ΔΔ
Garlic *(Allium sativum)* HT ΔΔ

For an elderly person with acute bronchitis:
Grindelia *(Grindelia robusta)* HT
Sweet Violet *(Viola odorata)* HT
Wild Cherry Bark *(Prunus Serotina)* HT

To stimulate blood circulation:
Cayenne *(Capsicum annum)* HT
Garlic *(Allium sativum)* HT ΔΔ

To relieve chest congestion and a wet cough:
Angelica *(Angelica archangelica)* HT ΔΔ
Cayenne *(Capsicum annum)* HT
Grindelia *(Grindelia robusta)* HT

To soothe a painful, harsh, and dry cough:
Horehound *(Marrubium vulgare)* HT ΔΔ
Marshmallow *(Althaea officinalis)* HT
Mullein *(Verbascum thapsus)* HT

To reduce mucus build-up in the lungs:
Cayenne *(Capsicum annum)* HT
Mullein *(Verbascum thapsus)* HT
Garlic *(Allium sativum)* HT ΔΔ

- Select one or more herbal tinctures. The herbal tinctures listed are synergistic combinations grouped according the patient's characteristics and symptoms. Use according to label instructions or add 10 to 30 drops to a half glass of water. Adjust dosage according to the patient's age and weight. For children under the age of six, use 10 drops. For children between ages six and twelve, use 15 to 20 drops. For older children, use 30 drops. Add essential oil/alcohol mixture as indicated above. Take the combined plant medicines on an empty stomach, three times per day before meals.

Suggestions: *Drink herbal teas and fresh, home-made juices. Use fresh citrus juices in moderation. Avoid caffeine, alcoholic beverages and citrus juices that have been either concentrated or pasteurized. Avoid dairy products and flavored yogurt. Eliminate products made with flour, including bread and pasta. Do not eat foods that contain chemical preservatives, flavorings, and additives. For coughing, mix the juice of one lemon to one teaspoon raw honey and swallow. You can also add the juice of four lemons to a quart of pure water. Add four teaspoons raw honey and stir. Sip slowly – do not drink. Sipping lemon water during two days will clear the throat.[6] If you have a chronic condition, avoid tobacco smoke completely. See a doctor if you have a hacking cough and another illness, if you are short of breath, or if you are coughing blood.*

ΔΔ Angelica HT: contraindicated if you are pregnant or if you have diabetes.

ΔΔ Bergamot EO: do not go into direct sunlight after using on skin.

ΔΔ Garlic HT: thins the blood. Consult with doctor before using if you are on anti-coagulant drugs.

ΔΔ Horehound HT: not for use by people with a heart condition.

ΔΔ Horsetail HT: contraindicated for pregnancy.

ΔΔ Thyme EO: contraindicated for thyroid disorder, high blood pressure, babies.

ΔΔ Wild Rosemary EO: contraindicated for epilepsy, high blood pressure, babies.

BUBONIC PLAGUE

Plague is a word once used to describe any widespread contagious disease associated with a high death rate. It exists in several different forms. Bubonic or oriental plague, also called pest, is an acute infection caused by the plague bacillus *Yersinia pestis*. It is commonly carried by fleas that infest rats and other rodents; for this reason rat control is an important preventive measure. Septicemic plague is characterized by massive infection of the blood stream. Some forms of plague, such as pneumonic plague, are transmitted directly from person to person, via infected droplets of sputum. Pneumonic plague is a highly virulent form of plague with extensive involvement of the lungs.

Bubonic plague runs a rapid, severe and often fatal course. The incubation period ranges from 2 to 10 days. Symptoms include high fever, restlessness, a staggering gait, mental confusion, exhaustion, delirium, shock, and coma. It begins with fever and chills, soon followed by headache, vomiting and sometimes, in the severe forms, by internal bleeding into the lungs, spitting of blood, breaking of small blood vessels on the skin (petechiae), and swelling of the lymph glands in the groin, armpits and neck. These swellings which may break down into ulcers and called buboes; hence the name bubonic plague. This disease was the black death that terrified Europe in the 14th century.

Pneumonic plague has an incubation period of 2 to 3 days. It is a sudden, severe illness with fever, chills, headache, cough with bloody sputum, and difficulty breathing. The skin develops a blue hue because with difficult breathing, less oxygen enters the body. If left untreated, pneumonic plague results in respiratory failure and certain death.

Plague is rare in North America, although occasionally it is found in ground squirrels and other wild rodents. It is common in some parts of Asia. If plague is accurately identified and treated with antibiotics at onset, it can be successfully cured. Patients should be quarantined for seven days and all members of the household should be treated under a physician's care. Antibacterial essential oils and herbs can be used as a support measure; they should target the lymphatic and respiratory systems and support the immune system.

DIRECTIONS FOR USE IN THE DIFFUSOR
Clove Bud *(Syzygium aromaticum)* *EO*
Lemon *(Citrus limon)* or **Lime** *(Citrus aurantifolia)* *EO*

- Add 20 drops Clove Bud to a 15 ml. bottle Lemon *(Citrus limon)* or Lime *(Citrus aurantifolia)* and use in an electric diffusor to disinfect the air.

DIRECTIONS FOR INTERNAL USE
Cinnamon Bark *(Cinnamomum zeylanicum)* *EO* ΔΔ
Clove Bud *(Syzygium aromaticum)* *EO*
Oregano *(Oreganum vulgare)* *EO* ΔΔ

- Internal use: Add 25 to 30 drops of each of the above essential oils to a 2-ounce bottle of brandy or vodka. Take 20–40 drops of EO/alcohol mixture along with 7–8 drops of each of the liquid herbals below:

Echinacea *(Echinacea angustifolia or E. purpurea)* *HT* ΔΔ
Elderberry *(Sambucus nigra)* *HT*
Garlic *(Allium sativum)* *HT* ΔΔ
Goldenseal *(Hydrastis canadensis)* *HT* ΔΔ

- Take the combined plant medicines 10 minutes before meals, three times per day.

Suggestions: *Plague is a risk factor associated with biological warfare. In the event of a plague epidemic, stay at home and do not venture out until health officials give the green light. If you have been exposed to plague, call your local health authorities immediately for instructions. Stay confined in your room to avoid exposing others. Wait until health authorities contact you with further instructions.*

ΔΔ Cinnamon Bark EO: contraindicated if you are pregnant.

ΔΔ Echinacea HT: avoid if allergic to ragweed.

ΔΔ Garlic HT: thins the blood. Check with doctor before using if you take on anti-coagulant drugs.

ΔΔ Goldenseal HT: do not use excessively (more than 3 times daily) or long term (longer than 7 days); contraindicated for pregnancy, hypertension, low blood sugar, allergy to ragweed.

ΔΔ Oregano EO: contraindicated for pregnancy.

CANDIDA ALBICANS

Candida albicans is a type of parasitic yeast-like fungus that inhabits the intestines, genital tract, mouth, esophagus, and throat. Normally this fungus lives in healthy balance with other bacteria and yeasts in the body. Certain conditions cause it to multiply, weakening the immune system and causing an infection known as candidiasis. The fungus can travel through the bloodstream to many parts of the body.

Candidiasis can affect many parts of the body. Most common are areas of the mouth, ears, nose, gastrointestinal tract, and vagina. There are many symptoms and illnesses that can result because of candidiasis; many are discussed in this book. They include diarrhea, colitis, abdominal pain, headaches, bad breath, rectal itching, impotence, memory loss, mood swings, prostatitis, canker sores, persistent heartburn, muscle and joint pain, sore throat, congestion, nagging cough, numbness in the face or extremities, tingling sensations, acne, night sweats, severe itching, clogged sinuses, PMS, burning tongue, white spots on the tongue and in the mouth, extreme fatigue, vaginitis, kidney and bladder infections, arthritis, depression, hyperactivity, a hypothyroid, adrenal problems, diabetes, athlete's foot, and jock itch.

Symptoms of candidiasis worsen in damp or moldy places and after the consumption of foods containing sugar and yeast.

When candida infects the vagina, it results in vaginitis characterized by a large amount of white, cheesy discharge and intense itching and burning (See Vaginitis). When the fungus infects the oral cavity, it is called thrush (See Mouth Infections). White sores may form on the tongue, gums, and inside the cheeks. In a baby, the white spots of oral thrush resemble milk spots. Oral thrush in a baby can spread to the mother's nipples by breastfeeding. Thrush may also affect the baby's buttocks, appearing as diaper rash.

Systemic candidiasis is an overgrowth of candida throughout the body.

Anyone having taken antibiotics often probably has an overgrowth of candida somewhere in the body. Antibiotics weaken the immune system and also destroy the friendly bacteria that normally keep candida under control. As it proliferates, the fungus releases toxins that damage the body further. Using corticosteroid drugs and birth control pills containing steroids also increase the chances of a fungal infection.

DIRECTIONS FOR INTERNAL USE

Oregano *(Oreganum vulgare)* *EO* ΔΔ

- Add 75–90 drops Oregano to a 2-ounce bottle Papaya tincture. Put 20–40 drops of this mixture into a half-glass warm water. Then add 10 to 15 drops of each of the following tinctures:

Black Walnut *(Juglans nigra)* *HT* ΔΔ
Pau d'Arco *(Tabebuia avellandedae)* *HT*

- Take the combined plant medicines 10 minutes before meals, three times per day.

Other useful essential oils: *Eucalyptus, Geranium, Patchouli, Rosewood, Sage, Savory, Sandalwood, Tea Tree, Thyme, Wild Rosemary.*
Other useful herbal tinctures: *Buchu, Cat's Claw, Elecampane, Garlic, Goldenseal.*
Suggestions: *For at least two to three weeks, eliminate all foods that contain yeast and sugar, including fruit. Also eliminate preserved foods, such as pickles and relishes. Eliminate or reduce using dairy products and carbohydrates (starchy foods). Substitute gluten-free grains, eating mainly raw or cooked vegetables, and slim cuts of meat,*

poultry, or fish. For further information about Candida Albicans and the Candida diet, please visit the web site www.healthpracticebooks.com to request a free, 10-page report provided electronically.

ΔΔ Black Walnut HT: contraindicated if you are pregnant.

ΔΔ Oregano EO: do not use if pregnant.

CHICKEN POX

Chicken pox is an acute viral disease characterized by mild symptoms including headache, fever, malaise and skin eruptions in successive "crops." Approximately 75 percent of all children get chickenpox by age 15, with epidemics more frequent in winter and spring. The illness is less common in adults. Chickenpox is caused by the herpes zoster virus, the same virus that causes shingles.

Chicken pox has an incubation period of two to three weeks. At onset, there's a slight elevation of temperature followed by eruptions on the back and chest within 24 hours. These eruptions continue to appear for a period of two to three days. Each crop requires 36 hours to pass through several stages.

Macules, colored spots of various colors, sizes and shapes, appear first. They then become *papules*, which are red, solid, circumscribed, and elevated areas of skin. Papules develop into vesicles, sac-like blisters which contain serous fluid. The final stage is crusting, where a scab or coat develops over the vesicle.

Because there are successive skin eruptions, the different forms may be found side by side in the same general location. The lesions are superficial and they tend to rupture very easily. After chickenpox subsides, there are some scars that usually remain as evidence of the attack.

INSTRUCTIONS FOR EXTERNAL APPLICATION
Lavender *(Lavandula augustifolia)* EO
Tea Tree *(Melaleuca alternifolia)* EO

- Spot treat the blisters with undiluted essential oils by dabbing with cotton swab. Do not rub or massage.
- Aromatherapy bath: add essential oils to 1 teaspoon (5 ml)

liquid soap and add to bath water. Follow these usage guidelines: babies 0–1 years, 1–2 drops essential oils; children ages 1 to 8, 2 to 4 drops essential oils; children 9 to 17, 6 to 8 drops essential oils; adults, 8–10 drops essential oils.[7]

- Inhalation: use EO in a diffusor during duration of treatment.

External use to relieve itching:
Peppermint *(Mentha piperita)* EO ΔΔ

- Dilute Peppermint essential oil with a carrier oil, using a 5% dilution. See p. 82 for dilution instructions. Apply where needed to relieve itching.[8]

DIRECTIONS FOR INTERNAL USE
Black currant *(Ribes nigrum)* HT
Burdock *(Arctium lappa)* HT ΔΔ

- Select one of the above herbal tinctures. Use according to label instructions or add 10 to 30 drops to a half-glass of water or juice, depending on child's age. If under the age of six, use 10 drops. For children between ages six and twelve, use 15 to 20 drops. For teens and adults, use 30 drops. Take three times per day, before meals.

Other useful essential oils: *Cypress, Eucalyptus, Geranium , Roman Chamomile.*
Suggestions: *Isolate the patient from others during contagious period (5 days prior to eruption and 6 days afterwards); avoid scratching the blisters. Keep the patients' fingernails trimmed. For dietary recommendations, see Scarlet Fever on p. 163. In case of reinfection or serious cases, see Shingles on p. 165.*

ΔΔ Burdock HT: may enhance the effect of insulin or blood sugar lowering medications.
ΔΔ Peppermint EO: contraindicated for pregnancy.

COLITIS
Inflammation of the colon, or colitis, is a frequently seen gastrointestinal disease. Colitis has many causes and can be called by

different names, such as spastic colon, spastic bowel, functional bowel disease, irritable colon, and irritable bowel syndrome, but not all of these names are technically correct. Colitis simply refers to an inflamed colon.

Symptoms of colitis include abnormal bowel movements, pain in the abdominal area, cramps, constipation alternating with diarrhea, gas, and mucus. Anemia, rectal bleeding, weight loss, and fever are not symptoms of colitis. When these accompany a change in bowel habits, see a physician.

Reliance on antibiotics leaves people vulnerable to frequent infections and reinfections from *staphylococcus, enteric bacilli, fungi,* and other types of microbes. Along with our weakened immune system defenses, the most common reasons for colitis are (1) fermentation and petrification of food in the colon resulting from a diet too rich in carbohydrates, starches, meats, eggs, and other foods that can ferment and petrify; (2) bacterial and viral attack, such as dysentery, shigella, and salmonella; and (3) parasitic invasion, including parasites, fungi, amoeba, and worms. Food allergies and lactose intolerance also play an important role.

Treating colitis involves lifestyle changes as well as eliminating the pathogens that cause infection. The lifestyle changes that are needed include more exercise, better diet, stress relief, and attitudinal changes. Eliminating pathogens involves removing the bacteria, viruses, parasites, and fungi that have developed in the colon. Essential oils and herbs are very useful, but they cannot resolve the problem unless the underlying causes are also addressed. Patients with colitis should seek help from a naturopath or an alternative health care provider.

The herbs and essential oils listed below are only a few among many that can be used in treating colitis. They can be used as a tonic to regulate the nervous system, to stimulate and calm the digestive tract, and to relieve symptoms such as constipation and diarrhea. Some plant medicines have very strong action, and overuse may cause problems.

When dealing with colitis, it is best to make lifestyle changes gradually and use a gentle approach.

To use plant medicines in treating colitis, match the needs and characteristics of the patient with the following herbs according to their medicinal properties.

INSTRUCTIONS FOR EXTERNAL APPLICATION
Lavender *(Lavandula augustifolia)* EO
Peppermint *(Mentha piperita)* EO ΔΔ

- External use: prepare a 5% dilution of essential oils in a carrier oil. See p. 82 for dilution instructions. Rub EO/carrier oil mixture clockwise on abdomen as often as needed.

DIRECTIONS FOR INTERNAL USE
Lavender *(Lavandula augustifolia)* EO
Peppermint *(Mentha piperita)* EO ΔΔ

- Add 20 drops of each of the above essential oils to a 2-ounce bottle Papaya tincture. Put 20–40 drops of this mixture into a half-glass warm water. Add 10 to 15 drops of each of the following tinctures:

Bilberry *(Vaccinium myrtillus)* HT ΔΔ
Gentian *(Gentiana lutea)* HT ΔΔ

- Take the combined plant medicines 10 minutes before meals, 3 times per day.

DIRECTIONS FOR INTERNAL USE
Herbal medicines should be administered according to the patient's needs and the medicinal effects desired. Select the essential oils and herbal tinctures that most closely match your needs. For best results, select 1 to 2 essential oils and also 1 to 2 herbal tinctures. Combine the selected plant medicines and use internally.

Plants that are anti-spasmodic:
Angelica *(Angelica archangelica)* HT ΔΔ
Lavender *(Lavandula augustifolia)* EO
German Chamomile *(Matricaria recutica)* EO
Orange *(Citrus sinensis)* EO
Peppermint *(Mentha piperita)* EO ΔΔ

Wormwood *(Artemisia absinthium)* HT △△

Plants that regulate Automatic Nervous System (ANS):
Gentian *(Gentiana lutea)* HT △△
Basil *(Ocimum basilicum)* EO △△
Thyme *(Thymus serpyllum)* EO △△

Plants to relieve constipation:
Black Walnut *(Juglans nigra)* HT △△
Fennel *(Foeniculum vulgare)* EO △△
Marshmallow *(Althaea officinalis)* HT
Orange *(Citrus sinensis)* EO
Slippery Elm *(Ulmus fulva)* HT

Plants to relieve diarrhea:
Black Walnut *(Juglans nigra)* HT △△
Carrot Seed *(Daucus carota)* EO
Geranium *(Pelargonium graveolens)* EO
Goldenseal *(Hydrastis canadensis)* HT △△

Digestive system tonics:
Lime *(Citrus aurantifolia)* EO
Bilberry *(Vaccinium myrtillus)* HT △△
Schizandra *(Schisandra chinensis)* HT △△

Plants that relieve tension, rapid heartbeat, increased blood pressure and sweating:
Blessed Thistle *(Cnicus benedictus)* HT
Lavender *(Lavandula augustifolia)* EO
Nutmeg *(Myristica fragrans)* EO △△
White Willow *(Salix alba)* HT △△

Essential oils that are antibacterial and antifungal:
Clove Bud *(Syzygium aromaticum)* EO
Lavender *(Lavandula augustifolia)* EO
Oregano *(Oreganum vulgare)* EO △△
Patchouli *(Pogostemon cablin)* EO
Sandalwood *(Santalum album)* EO

Suggestions: *See Diarrhea, p. 120. Drink fresh cabbage, carrot, or berry juice before breakfast. Avoid alcohol, coffee, and carbonated drinks. Eating cooked cabbage (including sauerkraut) is effective for colitis. Do not eat sausages or delicatessen meats often served with sauerkraut. Eliminate cheese, eggs, meats or other difficult to digest foods. Avoid vegetables with a lot of cellulose, such as celery, squash, or tomatoes; these may irritate the colon. Eat fruits apart from meals, chewing thoroughly. Replace white bread with whole-grain bread. Supplement with a multi-vitamin and mineral formula and extra magnesium.*

ΔΔ Angelica HT: contraindicated for pregnancy.

ΔΔ Basil EO: contraindicated for pregnancy.

ΔΔ Bilberry HT: contraindicated for diabetics.

ΔΔ Black Walnut HT: contraindicated for pregnancy.

ΔΔ Fennel EO: contraindicated for pregnancy, young children, and epilepsy.

ΔΔ Gentian HT: contraindicated for high blood pressure, ulcers.

ΔΔ Goldenseal HT: do not use excessively (more than 3 times daily) or long-term (longer than 7 days), contraindicated for pregnancy, hypertension, low blood sugar, allergy to ragweed.

ΔΔ Nutmeg EO: do not use if pregnant.

ΔΔ Oregano EO: do not use if pregnant.

ΔΔ Peppermint EO: contraindicated for pregnancy.

ΔΔ Schizandra HT: do not use if pregnant or nursing.

ΔΔ Thyme EO: contraindicated for pregnancy, thyroid disorder, high blood pressure.

ΔΔ White Willow HT: contraindicated for pregnancy, ulcers, allergy to aspirin. May cause nervousness, insomnia, headaches, convulsions.

ΔΔ Wormwood HT: contraindicated for pregnancy.

COMMON COLD

Coryza, or common cold, is an acute, catarrhal inflammation of the mucous membranes in the upper respiratory tract.

Many viruses can cause a cold. They are highly contagious. Symptoms include congestion of the nasal mucosa, watery discharge, nose sniffing and blowing, headaches, dull pains in the face and head, fever, body aches, tiredness, and feeling cold or chilly. Symptoms usually resolve within 5 or 10 days.

Colds are more likely to occur when people stay in overheated or dry rooms for a long period of time in winter. This affects the immune response, making developing a cold more likely. Cold, overheated, or moist feet, a damaged bronchial system, excessive use of antibiotics, unwanted physical or emotional stress, and aging are other conditions that increase susceptibility to colds.

INSTRUCTIONS FOR EXTERNAL APPLICATION

For topical application, bath, diffusor or steam inhalation:
Eucalyptus *(Eucalyptus globulus) EO*
Lavender *(Lavandula augustifolia) EO*
Tea Tree *(Melaleuca alternifolia) EO*

- Apply essential oils to the chest, back, and the bottoms of the feet. You may choose to use the essential oils neat, or dilute them with a carrier oil. Mix with a carrier oil at a 5% dilution (see page 82 for instructions).
- Aromatherapy bath: mix 6–8 drops of one or more of the above essential oils into a teaspoon bath gel or liquid soap. Dissolve under running water while soaking in the tub, 15–20 minutes, or use in the shower.
- Steam inhalation: for instructions, see p. 78.
- Diffusor: use Eucalyptus, Lavender, or Tea Tree in an electric diffusor to disinfect the air.

DIRECTIONS FOR INTERNAL USE

Oregano *(Oreganum vulgare) EO* ΔΔ
Thyme *(Thymus serpyllum) EO* ΔΔ

- Thyme is one of the best remedies for illnesses resulting from chill (influenza, head colds, stiffness, sore throat). If Thyme is not available, use Oregano. Take internally, 3 drops Thyme mixed in a spoon of raw honey, 3 times per day. If you prefer not using honey, prepare a formula using the essential oil mixed into vodka or brandy. Add 45 drops essential oil to a 2-ounce bottle alcohol. Take 20–40 drops of this mixture with a half-glass warm water or juice, three times per day before meals. If desired, you may use this together with the liquid herbals below.

Select one of the following synergistic combinations.
Cat's claw *(Uncaria tomatosa)* HT ΔΔ
Echinacea *(Echinacea angustifolia or E. purpurea)* HT ΔΔ
Elderberry *(Sambucus nigra)* HT

Burdock *(Arctium lappa)* HT ΔΔ
Marshmallow *(Althaea officinalis)* HT
Mullein *(Verbascum thapsus)* HT

- Select one to three herbal tinctures. Use according to label instructions or add 10 to 30 drops to a half-glass of water or juice. If taking two herbal tinctures, add 10 to 15 drops of each, and if taking three herbal tinctures, add 10 drops of each. Take 10 minutes before meals, three times per day.

Other useful essential oils: *Hyssop, Orange, Peppermint, Wild Rosemary.*
Suggestions: *See Influenza. Also see Bronchitis, Fever, Headaches, Muscle Aches and Pains, Sore Throat.*

ΔΔ Burdock HT: may enhance the effect of insulin or blood sugar lowering medications.
ΔΔ Cat's Claw HT: contraindicated for pregnant women, hemophiliacs, and organ transplant patients.
ΔΔ Echinacea HT: do not use if allergic to ragweed.
ΔΔ Oregano EO: contraindicated for pregnancy.
ΔΔ Thyme EO: contraindicated for pregnancy, thyroid disorder, high blood pressure.

CYSTITIS

Cystitis is inflammation of the bladder usually caused by bacterial infection. Symptoms include frequent and painful urination. The infection may spread from the urinary tract to the bladder and associated organs (kidney, prostate, urethra).

Cystitis is widespread among women. The infection is usually treated with antibiotics. According to Drs. Duraffourd, Lapraz, and Valnet, phytotherapy is "a heroic treatment" (i.e., very effective) for cystitis.[9]

If symptoms do not improve in a few days, or if there is pus or blood in the urine, consult with a physician. Medical supervision is also required to screen for renal calculus, structural defects (e.g., an obstruction of the urinary tract), or a prostate disorder.

INSTRUCTIONS FOR EXTERNAL APPLICATION

Lavender *(Lavandula angustifolia)* EO
Tea Tree *(Melaleuca alternifolia)* EO

- Apply Lavender or Tea Tree on lower abdomen, massage in a clockwise motion, three times per day or as often as needed.
- Add 10 drops Lavender or Tea Tree to two pints of water that has been boiled for disinfection then cooled for use with the oils, and apply directly to opening of urethra, using cotton swabs. Repeat several times per day, as often as possible, or each time after urinating.[10]
- Aromatherapy bath: Add 6–8 drops Tea Tree to a teaspoon liquid bath soap or shower gel, dissolve in bath water and use as a preventive measure.

DIRECTIONS FOR INTERNAL USE

Tea Tree *(Melaleuca alternifolia)* EO

- Take 2 drops Tea Tree essential oil internally in a gelatin capsule, every 20 minutes for four to six hours.[11]

—OR—

Cinnamon Bark *(Cinnamomum zeylanicum)* EO[12]
Clove Bud *(Syzygium aromaticum)* EO
Lavender *(Lavandula augustifolia)* EO
Oregano *(Oreganum vulgare)* EO △△

- For very resistant cases: Add 30 drops Cinnamon Bark, 5 drops Clove Bud, 5 drops Lavender, and 5 drops Oregano to a 2-ounce bottle of Papaya tincture. Put 40 drops of this mixture into a half glass of warm water, then combine with the herbal tinctures below:

Select one of the following synergistic combinations:

Bilberry *(Vaccinium myrtillus)* HT ΔΔ
Goldenrod *(Solidago virgaurea)* HT
Horsetail *(Equisetum arvense)* HT ΔΔ

—OR—

Bilberry *(Vaccinium myrtillus)* HT ΔΔ
Uva ursi *(Arctostaphylos uva ursi)* HT ΔΔ

- Select one or more (up to three) herbal tinctures. Use according to label instructions or add 10 to 30 drops to a half-glass of warm water. If taking two herbal tinctures, add 10 to 15 drops of each, and if taking three herbal tinctures, add 10 drops of each. Combine with EO/alcohol mixture. Take 5 times per day for the first 48 hours, then on following days, 3 times per day. Take 10 minutes before meals.

Other useful herbal tinctures: *Buchu, Couchgrass, Cranberry, Goldenseal, Marshmallow, Parsley, Slippery Elm.*
Other useful essential oils: *Bergamot, Black Pepper, Cedarwood Atlas, Frankincense, German Chamomile, Ginger Root, Lemon, Niaouli, Pine Tree, Thyme.*
Suggestions: *To control recurring urinary tract infections, purchase pH indicator strips at the pharmacy. Following directions on the box, check urine acidity. If urine is too acid, modify body-pH by drinking pear juice, lemon juice, or cranberry juice. You can also take cranberry capsules or tinctures. Use a good-quality multivitamin and mineral supplement. Reduce consumption of fatty meats, sugar, and sugary foods. Avoid using coffee, tea, and alcohol.*

ΔΔ Bilberry HT: contraindicated for diabetics.
ΔΔ Cinnamon Bark EO: avoid during pregnancy, do not apply undiluted to the skin.
ΔΔ Horsetail HT: do not use if pregnant.
ΔΔ Oregano EO: avoid during pregnancy.
ΔΔ Uva Ursi HT: contraindicated for pregnancy.

DIARRHEA

Diarrhea refers to frequent, abnormal passage of watery stool (bowel movement). Acute, infectious diarrhea is characterized by sudden onset. Accompanying symptoms include vomiting, cramping, thirst, and abdominal pain. People with IBS (irritable bowel syndrome) have diarrhea with intermittent constipation. Infantile diarrhea is characterized by dry skin, high temperatures, thirst, pains, and increase of stools with change in color and consistency.

Diarrhea can exist alone or can be a symptom of other problems. There are many possible causes, including bacterial and viral infection, intestinal parasites, food poisoning, allergies and food sensitivities, drinking contaminated water, caffeine, emotional tension and stress, and the use of certain drugs. People who travel may experience diarrhea as a result of infection by an enteropathic strain of *E. coli.*

Consult a health care provider if diarrhea continues for more than a few days. Diarrhea upsets the body's chemistry, resulting in low blood sugar, dehydration, and electrolyte imbalance. These conditions are especially dangerous in babies and infants. If a baby has five or more watery stools in a day, seek professional medical help.

INSTRUCTIONS FOR EXTERNAL APPLICATION
For children with diarrhea:
Roman Chamomile *(Chamaemelum nobile) EO*

- Mix 1 to 3 drops Roman Chamomile essential oil to one teaspoon carrier oil. Apply to a 6-month or older child. For older children, use 6 to 8 drops. Gently massage abdomen in a clockwise direction as often as needed.

DIRECTIONS FOR INTERNAL USE
For an adult with acute diarrhea:
Bilberry *(Vaccinium myrtillus) HT* ΔΔ
Clove Bud *(Syzygium aromaticum) EO*
Cypress *(Cupressus sempervirens) EO*
Roman Chamomile *(Chamaemelum nobile) EO*

- Add 30 drops of each of the above essential oils to a 2-ounce bottle Bilberry tincture. Take 20–40 drops of this mixture in a half-glass warm water, three times per day before meals.

Herbal tinctures for chronic diarrhea:
Astragalus *(Astragalus membranaceus)* HT

Herbal tinctures for acute diarrhea:
Red Raspberry *(Rubus idaeus)* HT
Purple Loosestrife *(Lythrum salicaria)* HT

Herbal tinctures for infectious diarrhea:
Black Walnut *(Juglans nigra)* HT ΔΔ
Lady's Mantle *(Alchemilla vulgaris)* HT
Purple Loosestrife *(Lythrum salicaria)* HT

- Select one or more (up to three) herbal tinctures. Use according to label instructions or, add 10 to 30 drops to a half-glass of water or juice. If taking two herbal tinctures, add 10 to 15 drops of each, and if taking three herbal tinctures, add 10 drops of each. Take 10 minutes before meals, three times per day.

Other useful herbal tinctures: *Bilberry, Goldenseal, Marshmallow.*
Other useful essential oils: *Black Pepper, Eucalyptus, Frankincense, Geranium, Ginger Root, Myrrh, Patchouli, Peppermint, Tea Tree, Thyme.*

ΔΔ Bilberry HT: contraindicated for diabetes.
ΔΔ Black Walnut HT: contraindicated for pregnancy.

EAR INFECTIONS

Ear infections can occur at any age, but small children often develop middle ear infections *(otitis media)* during colds. The eustachian tube, the drainage canal of the ear, is short and wide in infancy, increasing a child's susceptibility. Ear ache may also be linked to pain in the teeth or the jaws. Earache, teething, intolerance of pain are characteristic of infancy.

Ear infection can result in an abscess, pouring out pus and mucus. The accumulation of pus presses against the eardrum. This can cause pain, a sensation of fullness, fever, and temporary loss of hearing. Occasionally the pressure causes the pus to burst through the eardrum. When this happens, this does not mean that the infection has abated.

Recurrent ear infections are linked to a sugar-rich diet, which tends to depress the immune function. Another likely problem is a food allergy, such as an allergy or sensitivity to dairy products. Allergies cause the adenoids and tonsils to swell, blocking the eustachian tubes so that the ear does not drain and the ear canal becomes a breeding ground of bacteria. Doctors generally treat ear infections with antibiotics, but research shows that frequent reliance on antibiotics can increase the risk of frequent ear infections.[13]

INSTRUCTIONS FOR EXTERNAL APPLICATION

Geranium *(Pelargonium graveolens) EO*
Lavender *(Lavandula augustifolia) EO*
Tea Tree *(Melaleuca alternifolia) EO*

- Mix one to three of the above essential oils with a carrier oil. Use a 5% dilution (see p. 82). Gently massage mixture around the ear. Do not insert essential oils into the ear undiluted.
- Ear drops formula for a child: add 15 drops each of Lavender, Geranium, and Tea Tree essential oils to a 15 ml bottle of pure vegetable oil. The bottle will have 45 total drops essential oils and 360 drops carrier oil. Use 1–2 drops of this mixture into the ear canal every hour until the pain ceases. For the following week, use 1–2 drops three times per day. In the second week, use 1–2 drops one time per day. In the third week and weeks following, use 1–2 drops once per week.
- For an adult, use the same formula as above, doubling the number of EO drops.
- Lemon Juice Therapy: To prevent earaches from developing or in mild cases, try using 2 drops fresh lemon juice in each ear, morning and night, for 5 days.[14]

Useful herbal tinctures: *Garlic, Goldenseal, Mullein, Black Currant, Echinacea.*

Other useful essential oils: *Lemon, Niaouli, Roman Chamomile, Wild Rosemary.*
Suggestions: *Never use pins, nail files, or other hard objects to remove objects from the ear as this may scratch or perforate the eardrum. Eat foods rich in vitamins A, C, zinc or temporarily use these as supplements. Avoid dairy products or other allergenic foods, and reduce or eliminate the consumption of sugar.*

ECZEMA

Eczema is a common inflammatory disorder of the skin. It is characterized by redness and itching accompanied by oozing, crusting, and scaling.

Eczema is not a distinct disease but rather a sign or symptom of an underlying condition. An infection may come along or be superimposed over this. The medical literature suggests this may be a chronic infection caused by staph, strep, or a variety of fungi.[15]

Numerous factors can lead to eczema: genetic predisposition, imbalanced intestinal flora, leaky gut, food allergies, environmental contaminants, emotional stress, heat, increase in humidity, sweat, pets, hormone fluctuations, dust, molds, pollens, cosmetics and other personal care products, and wool clothing. Foods that can aggravate eczema include eggs, cow's milk, food coloring, tomatoes, fish, cheese, chocolate, and wheat.

Eczema is commonly treated using cortisone creams that may relieve symptoms and diminish eczema lesions. However, prolonged use of cortisone and corticosteroids can lead to problems. The body tends to accumulate fat in the abdomen, face and on the back of the neck. The immune system produces fewer disease-fighting antibodies, increasing the body's susceptibility to viral, bacterial, and fungal infections. Blood vessels near the surface of the skin become more visible, and the skin bruises more easily. Wounds heal more slowly, and blood pressure increases. The underlying conditions that lead to eczema are not addressed by using cortisone creams.

Essential oils are anti-inflammatory, antibacterial, antifungal, and can effectively reduce the swelling, itching, and scaling characteristic of eczema without undesirable side effects.

INSTRUCTIONS FOR EXTERNAL APPLICATION

Carrot Seed *(Daucus carota)* EO
German Chamomile *(Matricaria recutica)* EO
Tea Tree *(Melaleuca alternifolia)* EO

- If the area is small, apply one or more of the above essential oils directly to the affected area, without dilution. If the area is large, apply 3–6 drops of one or a combination of the above essential oils with a pearl-sized drop of carrier oil or lotion, as often as needed. The lotion should be free of harmful ingredients.
- Make the following eczema/psoriasis formula. Store in an amber-colored glass container. Apply directly to the skin often.[16]

  - 10 drops Bergamot *(Citrus bergamia)* EO ΔΔ
  - 10 drops German Chamomile *(Matricaria recutica)* EO
  - 20 drops Lavender *(Lavandula augustifolia)* EO
  - 20 drops Juniper Berry *(Juniperus Communis)* EO ΔΔ
  - 5 ml. Aloe Vera carrier oil
  - 5 ml. Sesame Seed carrier oil

DIRECTIONS FOR INTERNAL USE

Burdock *(Arctium lappa)* HT ΔΔ
Red Clover *(Trifolium pratense)* HT
Yellow dock *(Rumex crispus)* HT ΔΔ

- Select one or more (up to three) herbal tinctures. Use according to label instructions or, add 10 to 30 drops to a half glass of water or juice. If taking two herbal tinctures, add 10 to 15 drops of each, and if taking three herbal tinctures, add 10 drops of each. Take 10 minutes before meals, three times per day.

Other useful herbal tinctures: *Black Walnut, Calendula, Dandelion, Echinacea, Fumitory Root, Oregon Grape, Slippery Elm.*
Equally useful essential oils: *Bergamot, Cedarwood Atlas, Myrrh, Patchouli, Pine Needle, Sandalwood.*
Suggestions: *Consult with a health professional to determine the cause of your eczema. Develop a treatment plan accordingly. If your diet is deficient, supplement with*

the needed nutrients (especially B vitamins and essential fatty acids). If your problem is a food sensitivity, determine which foods to eliminate from your diet. Periodic fasting or the candida diet may be helpful to rid your body of toxins. See Candida albicans.

ΔΔ Bergamot EO: can irritate the skin when exposed to direct sunlight.

ΔΔ Burdock HT: may boost the effect of insulin or blood sugar lowering medications.

ΔΔ Juniper Berry EO: do not use if kidneys are infected or inflamed. Contraindicated for pregnancy.

ΔΔ Yellow Dock HT: may cause mild diarrhea or stomach upset in sensitive people.

EYE INFECTIONS

Eye infections are commonplace but must be taken seriously and treated promptly under medical supervision. Usually more than one part of the eye is infected. Untreated infection in one eye can spread to the other.

Infections that frequently affect the eyes include syphilis, gonorrhea, tuberculosis, measles, and scarlet fever. Reddened eyes, a mild form of conjunctivitis, usually accompanies upper respiratory infections. Infections that attack the interior of the eye are most damaging, but even those that enter the exterior surroundings of the eyeball can cause harm. Photophobia, the inability to look at light, is a common sign of an infection that has gone to the interior of the eye.

Blepharitis is an inflammation of the outer edges of the eyelids. It involves hair follicles and glands that open on the surface. Ulcerative Blepharitis is usually caused by bacterial infection; non-ulcerative blepharitis may be due to allergy, exposure to dust, smoke, or irritating chemicals. Symptoms include redness, itching, burning, and the feeling of having something in one's eye. Some people experience swelling of the eyelids, sensitivity to light, tearing, and loss of eyelashes. Crusts form that "glue" the eyes together during sleep. Styes and cysts may appear.

A *stye* is an infection of the lash roots and associated glands in the margins of the eyelids. It resembles a pimple or a boil along the course of a hair root. Styes usually come in crops and are often a sign of eyestrain and poor health. They usually soften in a day or two, discharging some infectious material before they are healed.

Conjunctivitis is an inflammation of the conjunctiva, the moist membranes that cover the white of the eye and line the upper and lower eye lids. The eyes appear swollen and bloodshot; they are often itchy and irritated. Because the infected membrane is often filled with pus, the eyelids tend to stick together after being closed for an extended period.

Pink eye is an epidemic form of conjunctivitis, and is highly communicable and contagious. It is usually caused by a specific germ, the *Koch–Weeks bacillus*. It may spread rapidly in a household or school by use of a common towel or possibly by hand-to-hand and hand-to-eye contact. Cleanliness is the key to protection against pink eye.

Trachoma is a chronic, contagious form of conjunctivitis, caused by a strain of *chlamydia trachomitis,* an organism closely related to *rickettsia.* The disease affects millions of people in Africa and Asia; it is also found in parts of the United States. More than 20,000,000 people have been blinded by this disease. Trachoma is sometimes called "granulated eyelids" because the infection causes severe scarring and turning out of the eyelids, which gives the eyes an ugly look. Surgery may be required when such eye lid deformities occur.

INSTRUCTIONS FOR EXTERNAL APPLICATION

Lavender *(Lavandula augustifolia) EO*

- To disinfect the external area around the eye, mix 3–5 drops Lavender with one teaspoon carrier oil. Carefully apply 1–3 drops of this mixture around the eyes. Do not apply essential oils into the eye itself. If this happens, rinse the eye with milk or a vegetable oil. Wipe out gently with a soft cloth or tissue.

Eye bright *(Euphrasia officinales) HT*

- Wash or dab the infected eye gently with a cool compress. A wash cloth applied to a stye can speed a stye coming to a head. You may pull out the hair around which the stye forms, but do not squeeze the stye as this may spread the infection.

Rose Hydrolat

- A hydrolat is the water that remains after plant distillation. Hydrolats are very healing yet gentle to the tissues. For eye infections and inflammation, Rose Hydrolat is highly recommended. Follow label directions.

DIRECTIONS FOR INTERNAL USE
Barberry *(Berberis vulgaris)* HT ΔΔ
Horsetail *(Equisetum arvense)* HT ΔΔ
Oregon Grape *(Berberis aquifolium)* HT ΔΔ

- Select one of the above herbal tinctures. Use according to label instructions or add 10 to 30 drops to a half glass water or juice. Take 10 minutes before meals, three times per day. You may also combine 15 drops Barberry with 15 drops Oregon Grape and use as instructed, in a half glass of water or juice before taking meals.

Other useful essential oils: *Clary Sage, Fennel, Geranium, German Chamomile, Roman Chamomile, Tea Tree.*
Suggestions: *To avoid spreading bacterial infection, use only sterile materials when working with the eye. Cleanliness is of the utmost importance. Temporarily avoid using eye makeup or mascara. Throw away previously used eye makeup brushes that may have become contaminated. Do not use cosmetics that contain harmful ingredients. If the eye infection does not clear up within 4 days, see a doctor.*

ΔΔ Barberry: contraindicated for pregnancy. Do not take internally for more than seven days.
ΔΔ Horsetail: contraindicated for pregnancy.
ΔΔ Oregon Grape: contraindicated for pregnancy.

FEVERS

Fevers are characterized by elevation of the body temperature above normal, a flushed face and hot, dry skin, headache, body aches, pain and discomfort, nausea and vomiting, constipation and sometimes diarrhea, and scant, deeply-colored urine. A fever is not an illness, but rather an indication that illness or disease may be present.

Fevers follow infectious diseases. As germs invade the body, immune-system cells release proteins that signal the body's heat-regulating centers, which are located in the hypothalamus. A fever is the body's defense, an attempt by the body to rid itself of microbes that cause harm. For this reason, a fever is usually helpful to overall health, and under normal conditions is no cause for concern.

In severe cases (usually a temperature over 105° F. or 40.5° C., but sometimes less) delirium may result from the elevated temperatures. Convulsions and coma are also risk factors, especially in children. In patients with cardiac problems, high fevers can cause irregular heart rhythms, chest pain, or heart attack. High fevers may cause birth defects during the first trimester of pregnancy. For fevers over 102° F. (or 103° F. in children) take steps to reduce fever and consult a health care provider.

If there is a stiff neck that is painful to move accompanying the fever, see a doctor immediately. (See "Suggestions" below.)

Use herbal tinctures according to their healing properties. Use the tinctures as long as the fever lasts, and up to 48 hours afterwards.

INSTRUCTIONS FOR EXTERNAL APPLICATION
Lavender *(Lavandula augustifolia) EO*
Roman Chamomile *(Chamaemelum nobile) EO*
Tea Tree *(Melaleuca alternifolia) EO*

- For a child or adult, disperse 3–5 drops essential oils in a bowl of water, dip wash cloth or sponge in mixture, sponge the patient down.
- Do not use any essential oils on a baby less than three months old unless you seek professional advice. For a baby up to three months old, use a sponge bath with water. Do not use rubbing alcohol. For a 3-month old or older baby, use only one drop of Lavender, Roman Chamomile or Tea Tree essential oil in a sponge bath.
- A full-body massage with Lavender can reduce fever quickly in an infant or young child. Mix 10 drops essential oils to 1 ounce

carrier oil and apply.

DIRECTIONS FOR INTERNAL USE (SYMPTOM RELATED)

Fever with little or no sweat; red, flushed face, rapid pulse; red tongue:
Yarrow *(Achillea millefolium)* HT

Fever with little or no sweat; dry, parched, red skin:
Elderberry *(Sambucus nigra)* HT

Fever with little or no sweat; dry skin, internal tissues and membranes are dry:
Pleurisy Root *(Asclepias tuberosa)* HT ΔΔ

Patient is an infant, has fever with little or no sweat:
Catnip *(Nepeta cataria)* HT

Fever with profuse sweating and perspiration:
Pleurisy Root *(Asclepias tuberosa)* HT ΔΔ
Lobelia *(Lobelia inflata)* HT ΔΔ
Elderberry *(Sambucus nigra)* HT

Low-grade fever, swollen glands, boils, signs indicating low immune response:
Calendula *(Calendula officinalis)* HT ΔΔ
Echinacea *(Echinacea angustifolia or E. purpurea)* HT ΔΔ
Goldenrod *(Solidago virgaurea)* HT

- Select one of the above herbal tinctures, depending the patient's symptoms. Use according to label instructions or add 10 to 30 drops to a half-glass of water or juice, depending on the age of the child. For children under the age of six, use 10 drops. For children between ages six and twelve, use 15 to 20 drops. For older children, use 30 drops. Take three times per day, before meals.

Other useful essential oils: *Black Pepper, Peppermint.*
Suggestions: *Never give aspirin to a child with a fever. Always see a health professional immediately if any of the following symptoms appear: a stiff neck that is painful to move; frequent, burning urination; blood in urine; severe headache and*

vomiting; watery diarrhea lasting more than 24 hours; swollen glands or rashes; shaking chills or chills alternating with sweating; pain focused in one area of the abdomen.[17] See Common Cold *(p. 115)* and Influenza *(p.143)*.

ΔΔ Calendula HT: do not take if you are taking drugs for anxiety or high blood pressure.

ΔΔ Echinacea HT: do not take if you are allergic to ragweed.

ΔΔ Lobelia HT: contraindicated for pregnancy. Can cause vomiting and other undesirable side effects.

ΔΔ Pleurisy Root HT: contraindicated for pregnancy.

GALL BLADDER INFLAMMATION

Cholecystitis, inflammation of the gallbladder, may be either an acute or chronic illness. Acute cholecystitis is usually caused by gallstones which block the bile duct. Bacterial infection or toxic chemicals that irritate can also cause inflammation. Symptoms of acute cholecystitis include fever, nausea, vomiting, and either a gradual or sudden pain in the upper abdomen which tends to move towards the back. In many cases, jaundice is visible. Because the condition can be life threatening, cholecystitis requires medical care.

Symptoms of chronic cholecystitis are similar to acute cholecystitis, but are less severe. Chronic cholecystitis may occur with or without gallstones. Not all patients with gallstones experience cholecystitis.

Phytotherapy can prevent the formation of gallstones through the use of *cholagogues* (herbs that stimulate the gallbladder to contract) and *choleretics* (herbs that stimulate the liver to secrete more bile). Antispasmodic herbs may also be used.

INSTRUCTIONS FOR EXTERNAL APPLICATION

Cinnamon Bark *(Cinnamomum zeylanicum) EO* ΔΔ
Lavender *(Lavandula augustifolia) EO*
Orange *(Citrus sinensis) EO* ΔΔ
Peppermint *(Mentha piperita) EO* ΔΔ
Wild Rosemary *(Rosmarinus officinalis) EO* ΔΔ

• Select one to three essential oils. Cinnamon Bark and

Lavender are antiseptic oils, capable of killing the germs that cause gallbladder inflammation. Peppermint and Wild Rosemary are cholagogues and choleretics. Nutmeg and Peppermint are believed capable of dissolving gallstones, although little scientific research has been done to verify this claim.[18] Orange is an antispasmodic essential oil.

- External use: Use a 5% dilution of essential oils mixed with a carrier oil (see p. 82.) Apply to the abdomen, over the gallbladder. The gallbladder is a pear-shaped organ that lies below the ribs, on the right side of the abdominal cavity below the liver.

DIRECTIONS FOR INTERNAL USE[19]
Nutmeg *(Myristica fragrans)* EO ∆∆
Marjoram *(Thymus mastichina)* EO
Wild Rosemary *(Rosmarinus officinalis)* EO ∆∆

- Add 7 drops of each of the above essential oils to a 2 ounce bottle Papaya tincture. Add 40–50 drops of this mixture to a half-glass of warm water. Then add 15 drops of each of the following herbs into the water:

Celandine *(Chelidonium majus)* HT ∆∆
Khella *(Ammi visnaga)* HT ∆∆

- Take combined mixture three times per day, 10 minutes before meals.
- Instead of Celandine and Khella, you may also use:

Fumitory Root *(Fumaria officinalis)* HT ∆∆
Gentian *(Gentiana lutea)* HT ∆∆
Madder root *(Rubia tinctorum)* HT ∆∆

Other useful herbal tinctures: *Artichoke, Burdock, Dandelion, Garlic.*
Other useful essential oils: *Lemon, Pine Needle.*
Suggestion: *Patients with an inflamed gallbladder should eat no solid food for a few days. At first only consume distilled water, and gradually add pear, apple, or beet juice*

over three days. Follow with a careful diet of shredded beets mixed with 2 tbs. olive oil, fresh lemon juice, and fresh, home-made apple sauce. Long term, eliminate fats from the diet and if overweight, begin a gradual weight-loss program.[20]

ΔΔ Celandine HT: do not exceed recommended dosage.

ΔΔ Cinnamon Bark HT: do not use undiluted on the skin. Avoid if pregnant.

ΔΔ Fumitory HT: laxative, do not exceed dosage. Do not use long-term.

ΔΔ Gentian HT: if you have high blood pressure, use with caution.

ΔΔ Madder Root HT: contraindicated for pregnancy.

ΔΔ Nutmeg EO: contraindicated for pregnancy; can cause hallucinations.

ΔΔ Orange EO: do not go into direct sunlight after applying on the skin.

ΔΔ Peppermint EO: do not use undiluted on the skin. Contraindicated for pregnancy.

ΔΔ Wild Rosemary EO: contraindicated for epilepsy, high blood pressure.

ΔΔ Khella HT: in sunlight, causes dermatitis in some people.

GASTRITIS

Gastritis is an inflammation or irritation of the inner lining (mucosa) of the stomach without an ulcer or sore being present. Common symptoms of gastritis include hiccups, loss of appetite, indigestion, pain or tenderness, nausea, vomiting, vomiting of blood, and dark stools. The electrolyte balance in body fluids becomes disturbed. *Atrophic gastritis* is a form of gastritis often found among the elderly, where stomach cells are destroyed, leading to pernicious anemia.

Enteritis, an inflammation of the small intestine, is often associated with colitis (See Colitis). Gastroenteritis is an inflammation of the stomach and small intestines, more particularly of the mucous tissues. It can be both a chronic or acute condition.

Bacterial infection, particularly the bacterium *Helicobacter pylori*, causes gastroenteritis. Other contributing factors include stress, poor diet, surgery, food poisoning, alcohol, and the use of certain medications (such as corticosteroids, NSAIDs, antibiotics, and cancer drugs). [21]

DIRECTIONS FOR INTERNAL USE

For gastritis in an adult: [22]

Roman Chamomile (*Chamaemelum nobile*) *EO*

Savory *(Satureja hortensis) EO* ΔΔ
Thyme *(Thymus serpyllum) EO* ΔΔ

- Add 7 drops of each of the above essential oils to a 2 ounce bottle Papaya tincture. Add 40 drops of this mixture to a half-glass of warm water. Then add 13 drops of each of the following herbs into the water:

Bilberry *(Vaccinium myrtillus) HT* ΔΔ
Blackberry *(Rubus fruticosus) HT*
Black Walnut *(Juglans nigra) HT* ΔΔ

- Take combined mixture three times per day, 10 minutes before meals.

Other useful herbal tinctures: *Artichoke, Calendula, Goldenseal, Marshmallow, Oregon Grape, Purple Loosestrife, Slippery Elm, Wormwood.*
Other useful essential oils: *Fennel, Ginger Root, Marjoram, Peppermint, Roman Chamomile.*
Suggestions: *Drink raw cabbage juice several times during the day. Reduce or eliminate consumption of alcohol, tobacco, coffee, tea, and caffeine.*

ΔΔ Bilberry HT: contraindicated for diabetics.
ΔΔ Black Walnut HT: contraindicated for pregnancy.
ΔΔ Savory EO: contraindicated for pregnancy.
ΔΔ Thyme EO: contraindicated for pregnancy, thyroid disorder, high blood pressure.

HEADACHES

Headaches often accompany an infectious disease, such as an infection of the sinuses, ears, eyes, nose or throat, or an infection in the digestive tract or the reproductive organs. Besides infections, there are many other causes of headaches.

Almost any disturbance in the body can cause a headache. Like poor immunity, headaches usually indicate the build-up of toxins in the body. A headache is a signal that the body is out of balance. If you have recurring headaches, it is important to find out why. Work with your health care practitioner to determine the root cause of the problem.

Herbal medicines are very effective against the pain and discomfort caused by headaches. The two plant remedies found below are effective to relieve most types of headache symptoms, including migraines. If you prefer not using them as herbal combinations, you can also use them as singles.

INSTRUCTIONS FOR EXTERNAL APPLICATION

Lavender (*Lavandula augustifolia*) EO
Helichrysum (*Helichrysum angustifolium*) EO
Peppermint (*Mentha piperita*) EO ΔΔ
Wild Rosemary (*Rosmarinus officinalis*) EO ΔΔ

- External use: mix the above essential oils with a carrier oil, using a 10% dilution (see p. 82). Apply blend to area of pain or across the forehead and temples. If the pain does not subside within ten minutes, apply Helichrysum and Lavender neat.
- If treating a child, massage the neck and shoulders using Lavender, apply neat.

DIRECTIONS FOR INTERNAL USE

Agrimony (*Agrimonia eupatoria*) HT
Celandine (*Chelidonium majus*) HT ΔΔ
Dandelion (*Taraxacum dens leonis or T. officinale*) HT ΔΔ
Licorice root (*Glycyrrhiza glabra*) HT ΔΔ

- Select one or more herbal tinctures. Use according to label instructions or add 10 to 30 drops to a half-glass of water or juice, depending on the age and weight of the child. Take the tinctures three times per day, before meals. Take 10 minutes before meals, three times per day.

ΔΔ Celandine HT: do not exceed recommended dosage.
ΔΔ Dandelion HT: do not use without doctor's permission if you have ulcers or gastritis.
ΔΔ Licorice Root HT: do not use if you have hypertension, liver disease,

diabetes, edema, rapid heart beat, or if you are taking dioxin-based drugs.
ΔΔ Peppermint EO: do not use undiluted on the skin. Avoid if pregnant.
ΔΔ Wild Rosemary EO: contraindicated for epilepsy, high blood pressure.

HEPATITIS

Hepatitis is an inflammation of the liver, often accompanied by jaundice (a yellow color in the eyes and skin). In some instances, there is enlargement of the liver. Hepatitis can lead to liver failure and death. The disease can result from viral infection, alcohol abuse, or exposure to toxic chemicals and drugs.

There are three different types of hepatitis: hepatitis A, B, and C. These viruses are genetically unrelated, but they cause similar symptoms.

The hepatitis A virus is spread very through fecal-oral transmission— particles from the stool of an infected person contaminates something another person puts in his mouth. Restaurant workers and others handling food should carefully wash their hands with a disinfectant soap after using the bathroom to avoid spreading hepatitis A.

Hepatitis A has an incubation period of two to six weeks. At onset of symptoms, the patient can experience jaundice, gastrointestinal and respiratory disturbances, enlarged and tender liver, muscle pain, itching, weight loss, nausea, fatigue, and spleen enlargement. The illness usually lasts less than two months. In a few cases, it can last up to six months.

Hepatitis B (also known as HBV) can be transmitted through contact with the blood or body fluids of an infected person. Symptoms are similar to those of hepatitis A. In many cases infected persons have no idea they are HBV carriers because there are no symptoms. However, they can still pass the illness on to others. Each year, an estimated 200,000 people in the U.S. develop HBV, resulting in 5,000 deaths annually.

The hepatitis C or HCV virus was not discovered until 1988. HCV spreads when the blood of an infected person enters another person's veins. Patients who received blood transfusions before 1992 are most likely to be infected. Prior to that year, screening procedures and standards for blood transfusions were more lax than they are today. Many people unwittingly received blood infected with the hepatitis C virus.

A person may have HCV without being aware of the infection. The illness has an extremely long incubation period, and it may take years before symptoms emerge. For the majority of HCV patients, the typical symptoms are only fatigue and mild depression. However, about 20 percent of HCV patients develop cirrhosis of the liver.

HCV can be spread through intravenous drug use and other unsafe practices. Some researchers believe that tattooing increases the risk of HCV. Nearly a third of HIV patients have HCV.

Regardless of the type of hepatitis, herbal medicine can be used to relieve symptoms, stimulate the immune system, and rebuild healthy liver cells.

DIRECTIONS FOR INTERNAL USE[23]
Wild Rosemary *(Rosmarinus officinalis) EO* ΔΔ

- Ingest 2 drops Wild Rosemary EO in a spoonful of honey. In addition, take 20 drops of each of the following herbal tinctures in water or juice:

Linden *(Tilia europa) HT*
Fumitory *(Fumaria officinalis) HT* ΔΔ
Black Walnut *(Juglans nigra) HT* ΔΔ

- Take three times a day before meals.

DIRECTIONS FOR INTERNAL USE
Lemon *(Citrus limon) EO*
Wild Rosemary *(Rosmarinus officinalis) EO* ΔΔ

- Add 20 drops of each of the above essential oils to a 2 ounce bottle Grapeseed oil. Add 40 drops of this mixture to a half-glass of warm water. Then add 15 drops of each of the following herbs to the water:

Dandelion *(Taraxacum dens leonis or T. officinale) HT* ΔΔ
Fumitory *(Fumaria officinalis) HT* ΔΔ
Madder Root *(Rubia tinctorum) HT* ΔΔ

- Take the combined mixture three times per day before meals. The length of treatment depends on the condition of the person.

Consult with your health care practitioner for advice.

Other useful herbal tinctures: *Agrimony, Artichoke, Barberry, Black Currant, Milk Thistle, Oregon Grape, Wormwood.*

Other useful essential oils: *Basil, Carrot Seed, Myrrh, Peppermint, Pine Needle.*

Suggestions: *Follow a low-fat or vegetarian diet. Avoid red meats, whole milk, palm kernel, coconut oil, margarine, shortening, safflower, corn, soy, and sunflower oils. Instead, use olive oil. Eat "bitter" greens such as dandelion, watercress, and mustard greens to stimulate bile flow and cleanse the liver. Also eat citrus fruits such as lemons and grapefruit. These fruits are rich in anti-oxidants, which are important for the health of the liver. Eliminate or reduce alcohol intake. Take nutritional supplements including lecithin, Vitamins B₁₂, C, and E.*

ΔΔ Black Walnut HT: contraindicated for pregnancy.

ΔΔ Dandelion HT: do not use without doctor's permission if you have ulcers or gastritis.

ΔΔ Fumitory HT: laxative, do not exceed dosage. Do not use long term.

ΔΔ Madder Root HT: contraindicated for pregnancy.

ΔΔ Wild Rosemary EO: do not use if you are an epileptic or have high blood pressure. Substitute Helichrysum EO or Grapefruit EO.

HERPES SIMPLEX

Herpes is an imprecise word that refers to vesicular eruptions caused by a virus infection. Cold sores, fever blisters, and genital herpes are caused by the herpes simplex virus. Shingles, also called zona, is caused by the herpes zoster virus, the same virus that causes chickenpox. See Shingles, (zona), p. 165.

Cold sores or fever blisters are blister-like sores which are usually found on the lips or face. Some people are particularly susceptible to cold sores, especially when their immune function is low or when they have been exposed to cold winds or hot sunshine. Cold sores are contagious and the infection can easily spread to other parts of the body or to other people.

Genital herpes is an infection transmitted by sexual contact. It affects both men and women. The skin of the genital region becomes red and itchy, and then small, painful blisters appear. These can last for several weeks. The first attack is generally the worst; however, reinfection is likely especially during times of stress, as a result of sexual activity, or as the result of another infection.

The herpes simplex virus usually attacks mucous membranes where they join the skin. They may also affect the gums of the mouth, the oropharynx area of the throat, and the eyes. See Eye Infections, p. 125, Mouth Infections, p. 155.

Cold sores, fever blisters, and genital herpes do not respond to antibiotics, but essential oils are effective because of their antiviral properties. Phytotherapy treatments must be sustained over a sufficiently long period of time to prevent reinfections.

INSTRUCTIONS FOR EXTERNAL APPLICATION
Essential oil blend for cold sores on the lips or face:
Cypress *(Cupressus sempervirens)* EO
Geranium *(Pelargonium graveolens)* EO
Lavender *(Lavandula augustifolia)* EO

- Spot treat, applying the essential oils directly to cold sores as soon as possible. Early intervention is important as this may prevent the blisters from developing altogether. Repeat treatment once per hour on the first day, thereafter less frequently for several days, until the condition has cleared.
- Aromatherapy bath for genital herpes: add 6–8 drops of the above essential oils to 1 teaspoon (5 ml.) liquid soap and add to running bath water. You may also use this as a douche to bathe infected body parts. This will soothe the skin and stop the infection from spreading.

DIRECTIONS FOR INTERNAL USE
Essential oil blend for herpes on the lips and face:[24]
Cypress *(Cupressus sempervirens)* EO
Lavender *(Lavandula augustifolia)* EO
Rose Otto *(Rosa damascena)* EO

- Add 7 drops of each of the above essential oils to a 2-ounce bottle Papaya tincture. Add 50 drops of this mixture to a half-glass warm water. Then add 16–18 drops of each of the following tinctures to the water:

Black Currant *(Ribes nigrum)* HT
Burdock *(Arctium lappa)* HT ∆∆
Plantain *(Plantago major)* HT

- Take the combined mixture before meals, three times per day. Follow this regime for one month.

For herpes affecting the mouth and gums:[25]
Geranium *(Pelargonium graveolens)* EO
Lemon *(Citrus limon)* EO
Savory *(Satureja hortensis)* EO ∆∆

- Add 30 drops Savory, 20 drops Geranium, and 15 drops Lemon to a 2-ounce bottle Papaya tincture. Add 50 drops of this mixture to a glass of apple juice. Also add 20 to 25 drops of each of the following tinctures to the juice:

Burdock *(Arctium lappa)* HT ∆∆
White Oak *(Quercus alba)* HT

- Take the combined formula 10 minutes before meals, three times per day.

Other useful herbal tinctures: *Astragalus, Black Walnut, Echinacea, Elderberry, Pau d'Arco.*
Other useful essential oils: *Bergamot, Eucalyptus, German Chamomile, Niaouli, Tea Tree.*
Suggestions: *Drink lemon juice or make the following drink: 1/4 part Cabbage juice, 1/4 part Black Currant juice, 1/2 part Apple juice. Drink this 3 times per day for 4 or 5 days, then once per day, in the morning, for three weeks.*[26] *Daily supplements—follow dosage recommendations on label: selenium; Vitamin A; Vitamin C; citrus bioflavonoids, zinc; L-Lysine and Lecithin. In case of genital herpes, also treat sexual partner in order to prevent reinfection. Abstain from sexual contact for at least a week during treatment.*

ΔΔ Burdock HT: may boost the effect of insulin or blood sugar lowering medications.

ΔΔ Savory EO: contraindicated for pregnancy.

HIV SUPPORT

The human immnodeficiency virus (HIV) destroys infection-fighting immune system cells, leaving the body open to attack from potentially fatal diseases. HIV infection has no symptoms at first, and may take ten years or longer to develop into Acquired Immune-Deficiency Syndrome (AIDS). Medical treatment for HIV may be effective in delaying the onset of AIDS, but this treatment is complicated and expensive, and cannot be provided to all patients.

In cases of HIV, the goal of phytotherapy is to improve the immune defense and prevent any new infections, particularly infections of the intestines and infections of the upper and lower respiratory tract. Intestinal infections are very frequent in HIV-positive patients and can lead to weight loss, a sign that the infection is becoming worse. Infections of the respiratory tract, especially pulmonary infections, greatly aggravate the general condition of the patient and create concerns about tuberculosis.

INSTRUCTIONS FOR EXTERNAL APPLICATION
To boost the immune system and prevent pulmonary infection:
Hyssop *(Hyssopus officinalis)* EO ΔΔ
Niaouli *(Melaleuca viridflora)* EO

- Apply the above essential oils in an aromatherapy bath at least two times per week. Mix 6–8 drops of essential oils into a teaspoon of bath gel or liquid soap. Dissolve under running water while soaking in the tub, 15–20 minutes, or use in the shower. In addition, mix 6–8 drops essential oils with one teaspoon carrier oil, rub on bottoms of the feet, or use in a massage.

DIRECTIONS FOR INTERNAL USE
To prevent intestinal infection:
Cinnamon Bark *(Cinnamomum zeylanicum)* EO ΔΔ

Lavender *(Lavandula augustifolia) EO*
Oregano *(Oreganum vulgare) EO* ΔΔ

- Select one to three of the above essential oils. Mix 45 drops essential oils (15 of each kind) into a 2-ounce bottle vodka or brandy. Add 20 to 40 drops of this mixture to a half-glass water or juice. Take three times per day, before meals. Use occasionally as a preventive measure, not for everyday use or longer than three weeks.

Tritherapy with essential oils:
Cinnamon Bark *(Cinnamomum zeylanicum) EO* ΔΔ
Eucalyptus *(Eucalyptus globulus) EO*
Wild Rosemary *(Rosmarinus officinalis) EO* ΔΔ

- According to L. Hervieux, M.D., "For a fairly moderate cost, this therapy can be adapted as a basic treatment for each patient and prescribed more aggressively for acute patients, to treat overall tone, immunity, bowel elimination and as an antibacterial, improving the patient's mental health. Patients will find that this therapy provides much-appreciated daily relief which can be prescribed in conjunction with traditional therapies." [27]

Herbal tinctures for HIV support:
Astragalus *(Astragalus membranaceus) HT*
Cat's Claw *(Uncaria tomatosa) HT* ΔΔ
Licorice Root *(Glycyrrhiza glabra) HT* ΔΔ
Lomatium *(Lomatium dissectum) HT* ΔΔ

- Take Astragalus, Cat's Claw, Licorice Root, or Lomatium as singles. Combining these may not result in a synergistic blend; scientific information has not been published. Consult with your health care practitioner for instructions, or select one of the tinctures. Use according to label instructions or add 10 to 30 drops to a half glass of water or juice. Take 10 minutes before meals, three times per day.

Suggestions: *See Bronchitis, Gastritis.*

ΔΔ Cat's Claw HT: contraindicated for hemophiliacs, organ transplant patients, and pregnancy.

ΔΔ Cinnamon Bark EO: contraindicated for pregnancy. Avoid using undiluted on the skin.

ΔΔ Hyssop EO: contraindicated for pregnancy, epilepsy.

ΔΔ Licorice Root HT: do not use if you have diabetes, edema, hypertension, liver disease, rapid heart beat, or if you take dioxin-based drugs.

ΔΔ Lomatium HT: blood thinner, if you're on anti-coagulant medication, check with your doctor before using. Do not take in large doses.

ΔΔ Oregano EO: contraindicated for pregnancy.

ΔΔ Wild Rosemary EO: do not use if you are an epileptic or have high blood pressure. Substitute Helichrysum EO or Grapefruit EO.

IMPETIGO

Impetigo is a highly contagious bacterial skin infection that occurs most often in children. The face is the primary region affected, especially in the area of the mouth and nostrils. The neck, hands, or knees are other areas where pustules may appear. It starts as a reddish discoloration but soon develops into blisters and a yellowish crust. The pustules sometimes burst, releasing a highly infectious solution. If carelessly touched, the infection can spread to other parts of the body. Occasionally, it becomes a systemic condition requiring medical treatment.

INSTRUCTIONS FOR EXTERNAL APPLICATION

Geranium (*Pelargonium graveolens*) *EO*
Lavender (*Lavandula augustifolia*) *EO*
Niaouli (*Melaleuca viridflora*) *EO*

• External application: select one to three essential oils. Using the tip of a cotton swab, apply 2–3 drops essential oils directly to small areas of the body. Repeat twice daily. Do not allow anything to touch the cotton swab after it has been used. Throw it away.

• To promote cleanliness and to disinfect the air, use the diffusor and the aromatherapy bath. See Bronchitis (p. 102) for instructions.

DIRECTIONS FOR INTERNAL USE
For an adult with a systemic infection:
Oregano *(Oreganum vulgare)* EO △△

- For an adult with a systemic infection: Add 45 drops Oregano to a 2-ounce bottle vodka or brandy. Take 20 to 40 drops of this mixture in a half-glass warm water or juice, three times per day before meals.

Other useful essential oils: *German Chamomile, Oregano, Savory, Tea Tree, Thyme.*

Suggestions: *Do not use non-steroidal, anti-inflammatory drugs (NSAIDs) such as aspirin or ibuproven. These drugs suppress the immune response and increase the risk of systemic infection.*

△△ Oregano EO: contraindicated for pregnancy.

INFLUENZA

Influenza or flu is a highly contagious viral illness that attacks the respiratory system. Symptoms include sudden onset, fever, chills, headache, muscle pain or tenderness, and sometimes physical or nervous exhaustion.

Influenza is usually more prevalent in winter and spring. It is spread by discharges from the mouth and nose of infected persons.

The illness has an incubation period of between one and three days. It usually begins suddenly, with malaise, chilliness, severe pain in the head or back, and fever. Sneezing, cough, hoarseness, symptoms of the common cold, and various intestinal complaints may manifest. It usually runs its course in four to five days, but some people experience lassitude for weeks or months after the acute phase disappears.

Influenza may result in secondary complications, such as bacterial infection of the nasal sinuses, middle ear, and lungs.

The influenza virus has shown great genetic variation, which accounts for the frequent epidemics among those who have been previously exposed to influenza caused by different strains of the virus.

DIRECTIONS FOR INTERNAL USE
Flu formula for internal use:[28]

Cypress (*Cupressus sempervirens*) EO
Tea Tree (*Melaleuca alternifolia*) EO
Thyme (*Thymus serpyllum*) EO ΔΔ
Wild Rosemary (*Rosmarinus officinalis*) EO ΔΔ

- Add 8 drops Cypress, 8 drops Tea Tree, 5 drops Thyme, and 5 drops Wild Rosemary into a 2-ounce bottle brandy or vodka. Add 40 drops of this mixture to a half-glass warm water. Also add 13 drops of each of the following tinctures to the water:

Artichoke (*Cynara scolymus*) HT ΔΔ
Black currant (*Ribes nigrum*) HT
Horsetail (*Equisetum arvense*) HT ΔΔ

- Take the combined mixture 10 minutes before meals, three times per day.

Alternative flu formula for internal use:
Cinnamon Bark (*Cinnamomum zeylanicum*) EO ΔΔ
Lavender (*Lavandula augustifolia*) EO
Tea Tree (*Melaleuca alternifolia*) EO
Pine Needle (*Pinus sylvestris*) EO

- Mix 8 drops of each of the above essential oils into a 2-ounce bottle brandy or vodka. Add 40 drops of this mixture to a half-glass warm water. Also add 20 drops of each of the following tinctures to the water:

Elecampane (*Inula helenium*) HT ΔΔ
Horsetail (*Equisetum arvense*) HT ΔΔ

- Take the combined mixture 10 minutes before meals, three times per day.

Suggestions: *Patients with influenza require 24–48 hours bed rest, a well-balanced diet, and liquids. The diet should include foods rich in magnesium, such as green leafy vegetables, tofu, lemon, brown rice, and wheat germ. The best liquids are natural fruit* *juices rich in Vitamin C, including fresh, homemade lemonade. Other recommended liquids include water, vegetable bouillon, soups and herbal teas. You can make a "hot toddy" by adding 1 clove and 1 piece cinnamon stick to 4–6 cups of water. Boil the water for 3 minutes, and then let stand for 20 minutes to infuse. Add a sprig of thyme, some lemon juice, and lavender honey to sweeten. Drink this mixture hot, 2 to 4 cups per day, for 2 to 5 days.[29] Use the diffusor with Lemon, Eucalyptus, Lavender or another suitable essential oil to disinfect the air and to help keep nasal passages clear. See Common Cold, p. 115; Fever, p. 127; Sore Throat, p. 169. In the case of "stomach flu" or "intestinal flu" please see Gastritis, p. 132. If there is diarrhea, see Diarrhea, p. 120.*

ΔΔ Artichoke HT: Do not use if you are pregnant, have gallbladder disease, gallstones, liver disease, kidney disease, or if you're allergic to plants in the Asteraceae family.

ΔΔ Cinnamon Bark EO: contraindicated for pregnancy. Do not use undiluted on the skin.

ΔΔ Elecampane HT: contraindicated for pregnancy.

ΔΔ Horsetail HT: contraindicated for pregnancy.

ΔΔ Thyme EO: contraindicated for pregnancy, thyroid disorder, high blood pressure.

ΔΔ Wild Rosemary EO: contraindicated for epilepsy and high blood pressure.

INTESTINAL PARASITES AND WORMS

A parasite is an organism that lives in or on another organism in order to obtain its nutrients. Parasites infest the intestinal tract and other body cavities of the host and can cause disease by infesting cells or directly destroying them. There are different types of parasites, for example, large parasites or pathogenic animals, which include nematodes, insects, worms, flukes, and snails, and small parasites, single-cell organisms larger than bacteria, such as protozoa and amoeba.

Large parasites are usually large enough to be seen by the naked eye. Their size can range from less than an inch to more than 12 inches long. Large parasites inhabit the intestinal tract and usually stay there. In contrast, small parasites are microscopic in size. Small parasites can travel in the bloodstream and infect any part of the body.

Adult tapeworms come from eating raw, undercooked, or infected meat. Adult worms can reach a length of more than 15 feet in the digestive tract.

Enterobius is a parasitic nematode worm (a pinworm) that is frequently found in children. Pinworms are very infectious and can cause itching in the anal area.

Giardia lamblia is a protozoan found in the water of rivers, streams, and lakes. When hunters, backpackers and fishermen make the mistake of drinking this water without boiling, they can contract *giardiasis*, which causes diarrhea, nausea, weight loss, and weakness.

Medical tests are available that can identify certain parasites. But many parasites cannot be identified through medical testing, primarily because of the overwhelmingly large number and variety of different parasites.

Low energy, skin rashes, pains, frequent colds, flu, constipation, or other chronic conditions can indirectly indicate the presence of parasites. The reason is simple: parasites live off the body and use the body's nutrients. In addition, they secrete toxins which compromise the immune system. Certain parasites cause arthritic conditions by getting into joints and eating the calcium lining of bones.

Many essential oils are vermifuges, agents for expelling parasites and intestinal worms. The French doctors primarily use essential oils in the treatment of intestinal parasites, but herbs are also effective.

INSTRUCTIONS FOR EXTERNAL APPLICATION
Basil *(Ocimum basilicum)* *EO* ΔΔ
Cinnamon Bark *(Cinnamomum zeylanicum)* *EO* ΔΔ
Oregano *(Oreganum vulgare)* *EO* ΔΔ

- Mix 6–8 drops essential oils with a teaspoon carrier oil, massage on abdomen in a clockwise direction, or apply to bottoms of feet.

DIRECTIONS FOR INTERNAL USE
For a child or adult with a systemic parasitic infection:[30]
Basil *(Ocimum basilicum)* *EO* ΔΔ
Cinnamon Bark *(Cinnamomum zeylanicum)* *EO* ΔΔ
Oregano *(Oreganum vulgare)* *EO* ΔΔ

- Mix 15 drops of Basil, 15 drops Oregano, and 10 drops Cinnamon Bark with a 2-ounce bottle of Grapeseed oil. Swallow 10 to 30 drops of this mixture using a half-glass warm water or vegetable capsules. Adjust dosage according to the patient's age and weight. For children under the age of six, use 10 drops. For children between ages six and twelve, use 15 to 20 drops. For older children and adults, use 30 drops. Take three times per day before meals, for six weeks.

As an alternative to using essential oils, use herbal tinctures:
Black Walnut *(Juglans nigra)* HT ΔΔ
Cascara Sagrada *(Rhamnusd purshiana)* HT ΔΔ
Garlic *(Allium sativa)* HT ΔΔ

- Select one or more (up to three) herbal tinctures. Use according to label instructions or, add 10 to 30 drops to water or juice. If taking two herbal tinctures, add 10 to 15 drops of each, and if taking three herbal tinctures, add 10 drops of each. Take 10 minutes before meals, three times per day, for six weeks.

Other useful herbal tinctures: *Elecampane, Gentian, Goldenseal, Oregon Grape, Pau d'Arco.*
Other useful essential oils: *Caraway Seed, Eucalyptus, Geranium, Lavender, Roman Chamomile.*
Suggestions: *Treat all members of the family at the same time as the person with parasites. Personal hygiene is very important. Disinfect underwear, towels, and bed linens. Cut and clean fingernails and keep hands clean. Drink 1/2 cup raw cabbage juice in the mornings before breakfast, for 15 days.*[31]

ΔΔ Basil EO: contraindicated for pregnancy.
ΔΔ Black Walnut HT: contraindicated for pregnancy.
ΔΔ Cascara Sagrada HT: contraindicated for pregnancy.
ΔΔ Cinnamon Bark EO: contraindicated for pregnancy. Do not use undiluted on the skin.
ΔΔ Garlic HT: Thins the blood. If you use anti-coagulant drugs, consult with a doctor before using.
ΔΔ Oregano EO: contraindicated for pregnancy.

KIDNEY INFECTION

Pyelonephritis is an inflammation of the pelvis and kidney, the result of a microbial attack. The infection is marked by a sudden onset of chilliness and fever, with a dull pain in the flank over either or both kidneys. The kidneys feel tender to the touch. Usually, symptoms are similar to those of cystitis: burning urgency and frequent urination.

INSTRUCTIONS FOR EXTERNAL APPLICATION

Fennel *(Foeniculum vulgare) EO* ΔΔ
Ginger Root *(Zingiber officinale) EO*
Helichrysum *(Helichrysum angustifolium) EO*

- Mix 6–8 drops of one or more of the above essential oils with a teaspoon of carrier oil, massage over the kidneys or bottoms of feet.

DIRECTIONS FOR INTERNAL USE[32]

Lavender *(Lavandula augustifolia) EO*
Pine Needle *(Pinus sylvestris) EO*

- Mix 45 drops of each of the above essential oils into a two-ounce bottle Papaya tincture. Add 40 drops of this mixture to a half-glass warm water. Also add into the water 20 drops of each of the following tinctures:

Bilberry *(Vaccinium myrtillus) HT* ΔΔ
Goldenrod *(Solidago virgaurea) HT*

- Take the combined mixture three times per day, before meals.

Other useful herbal tinctures: *Buchu, Khella, Garlic, Juniper, Uva Ursi.*
Other useful essential oils: *Cinnamon Bark, Oregano, Pine Needle, Sandalwood, Thyme.*
Suggestions: *see Cystitis, p. 117.*

ΔΔ Bilberry HT: contraindicated for diabetics.
ΔΔ Fennel EO: contraindicated for pregnancy, young children, epilepsy.

LICE INFESTATION

Lice are small, wingless insects. They have a predilection for humans, and can infest the hair, body, and clothing. Human lice are the primary transmitters of epidemic typhus, trench fever, and relapsing fever. They also transmit plague.

Pediculosis capitis refers to an infestation with head lice. Itching causes people to scratch their heads. The scratches then become inflamed as bacteria invade. Pustules, crusts, and suppurations resembling eczema appear. The hair has a matted appearance and gives rise to an unpleasant odor. The majority of victims are children attending public schools; however, adults can be victims as well.

Pediculosis corporis refers to an infestation of body lice. Body lice ("cooties") live primarily in or on clothing. The lice suck blood from the body, leaving only a tiny bite of pin-point size. After a week or so, these bites begin to resemble hives. The result is intense itching. In severe cases, large patches of skin turn red, and victims complain of feeling weak, tired, and irritable. A mild fever may accompany this illness.

Pediculosis pubis is an infestation of crab lice, usually in the pubic region. They can also be found in the beard, in eyebrows, and in eyelashes. Hairy individuals can sometimes find them on their body surface. Crab lice can be acquired through sexual relations, by wearing contaminated clothing, from toilet seats, or from bed clothes. In light-skinned individuals, blue-gray spots can sometimes be found in the genitals.

Lice infestations are far more common than is generally supposed. If one member of the family has head lice, this can easily spread to the whole family. If one person in a family has head lice, treat all family members for head lice.

Garlic tincture can be used as a preventive measure against lice. Essential oils can kill lice but they are ineffective against the eggs laid by lice.[33]

INSTRUCTIONS FOR EXTERNAL APPLICATION
Lavender *(Lavandula augustifolia)* EO
Lemon *(Citrus limon)* EO ΔΔ
Tea Tree *(Melaleuca alternifolia)* EO

- Select one to three of the essential oils listed. For head lice, mix 6–8 drops essential oils to a teaspoon shampoo or conditioner. Wash hair thoroughly and let stand for 5 to 10 minutes, then rinse. Continue treatments daily until you are certain that all eggs laid by the lice have finished hatching. For body lice, add 6–8 drops essential oils to a teaspoon liquid soap. Wash all body regions except the eyes and the genitals to avoid irritating sensitive tissues. (If burning occurs, do not apply water. Essential oils do not mix with water. Instead, use milk or a vegetable oil.)

- For crab lice in the genitals: add 1–2 drops essential oils to a teaspoon of liquid soap. Gently wash the affected area. Discontinue use if there is irritation.

- For a clothing antiseptic, add 8–10 drops Oregano essential oil to 1/4 cup liquid soap and wash gently. Rinse thoroughly. If using a washing machine to wash clothing or bedding, add 20–30 drops Oregano essential oil to the wash cycle.[34] Use hot water for the wash cycle followed by drying in a drying machine set at hot.

Garlic (*Allivum sativum*) HT ΔΔ

- Take Garlic as a preventive measure: use according to label instructions or, add 10 to 30 drops to water or juice. Take three times per day before meals.

ΔΔ Garlic HT: thins the blood. If you use anti-coagulant drugs, consult with a doctor before using.

ΔΔ Lemon EO: do not go into direct sunlight after applying on the skin.

LYME DISEASE

Lyme disease is a bacterial infection spread by ticks traveling with deer, mice, and other animals. It is the most common tick-born illness in the United States.[35]

The illness was first named in 1976, when a cluster of cases were reported in Lyme, Connecticut, USA. The ticks fall from animals into brush and are then picked up by people passing by. Pets such as dogs and cats can also pick them up and transmit them to humans. Fortunately, most ticks do not carry the bacteria *Borrelia burgdorferi*, which causes Lyme disease.

The ticks are quite small, roughly the size and color of poppy seeds. They are difficult to spot. At least half of all tick bites are not noticed at all because the bite is painless. Ticks fall from the body after feeding for several days. Once the tick begins to feed, bacteria can be transferred to its host. The longer the feeding, the greater the risk of infection.

Diagnosing Lyme disease can be difficult, because the symptoms resemble other illnesses such as flu, gout, chronic fatigue syndrome, lupus, and multiple sclerosis. A blood test has been developed to identify Lyme disease. The test measures the number of antigens present in the blood in the days following infection.

A rapidly expanding red rash, three or four inches across, is a symptom of Lyme disease. It is circular in shape and resembles a bull's eye. This is accompanied by symptoms of cold or flu: aches, pain, swollen glands, fever, headache, and general malaise.

In days or weeks following infection, patients develop muscle and joint pain with redness affecting the knees and other large joints. In 10 percent of cases, patients develop chronic arthritis. If left untreated, 15 percent of patients develop meningitis or nerve pain.

The earlier Lyme disease is diagnosed and treated, the greater the chances of a cure.

INSTRUCTIONS FOR EXTERNAL APPLICATION
Oregano *(Oreganum vulgare)* *EO* ΔΔ

- External use: Oregano kills ticks. Saturate a cotton ball with Oregano, then apply to the location of the bite. After the tick is dead, gently remove it, using tweezers if necessary. Seek medical help.[36] After removal of the tick, continue dabbing the affected area for 2–3 days with Lavender or Tea Tree essential oil.

Note: do not try to burning the tick out using a match or using home remedies such as kerosene or petroleum jelly. If using tweezers, do not twist the tweezer as you pull, and do not squeeze the tick's body. Otherwise, you may unwittingly inject bacteria into the skin. After removal, save the tick in a small bottle or jar so you can take it to the doctor for identification.

<u>DIRECTIONS FOR INTERNAL USE</u>
Oregano *(Oreganum vulgare)* EO ΔΔ

• Internal use: if you suspect a tick infection, immediately mix 90 drops Oregano essential oil to a 2 ounce bottle vodka or brandy. Take 20–40 drops of mixture in a glass of water or juice. Use as needed, not for every day use longer than three weeks.

Teasel *(Dipsacus sylvestris)* HT

• Naturopath Matthew Wood reports a high rate of success with Teasel *(Dipsacus sylvestris)* in treating patients with Lyme Disease.[38] Use according to label instructions.

Other useful herbal tinctures: *Echinacea, Dandelion, Goldenseal, Horsetail.*
Other useful essential oils: *Cinnamon Bark, Clove Bud, Frankincense, Lavender, Peppermint, Tea Tree.*
Suggestions: *For flu-like symptoms, see Common Cold, p. 115; Influenza, p. 143. For pain in the joints, see Muscle Aches and Pains, p. 159. As a preventive measure, before going into the woods and field, apply insecticide essential oils to body and clothes. For instructions, see p. 100. After spending time outdoors, immediately check yourself carefully for ticks or tick bites. Look for small raised bumps or pinpoint-size specks on clothing. If children have been outdoors during the summer or fall, look closely at their hair, ears, underarms, legs, and trunk. Have them shower when they come in, and wash their clothes immediately. Then dry the clothes for half hour in an electric clothes dryer. Washing clothes will notnecessarily kill ticks, even if you use hot water and bleach.*

ΔΔ Oregano EO: contraindicated for pregnancy, do not use undiluted on the skin.

MEASLES

A highly contagious disease marked by skin eruptions over the entire body, fever, malaise, watery eyes, sneezing, nasal congestion, and a barking cough. Koplik's spots, white spots resembling grains of sand, may appear on the mucous membranes of the mouth. Measles is caused by the rubeola virus. It is most common among school children with outbreaks occurring in the winter and spring.

Measles has an incubation period lasting from 10 to 20 days. Onset is gradual. Initial symptoms include symptoms of the common cold, inflammation of the nasal passages, drowsiness, loss of appetite, and a gradual elevation of temperature. On the second or third day, Koplik's spots develop in the mouth, opposite the molars. Eyes sensitive to light and coughing comes next, and the body's high temperature recedes somewhat. On the fourth day, the fever increases again and a rash appears on the face, giving it a swollen, mottled appearance. The rash then extends to other areas of the body.

In strong, well-nourished children the prognosis for recovery from measles is usually very good. However, measles can result in grave complications. Always consult a doctor. Phytotherapy shortens the duration and intensity of the attack.

INSTRUCTIONS FOR EXTERNAL APPLICATION
Cypress (*Cupressus sempervirens*) *EO*
Eucalyptus (*Eucalyptus globulus*) *EO*

- For topical application, select one or both essential oils. Mix with a carrier oil at a 2% dilution and apply to the chest, back, and the bottoms of the feet. Instead of diluting, you may choose to use Lavender or Tea Tree EO neat. (For instructions on preparing dilutions, see p. 82.)
- Inhalation: Use steam inhalation to soothe coughing. See Common Cold, p. 115.

Air antiseptic:
Lavender (*Lavandula augustifolia*) *EO*
Lemon (*Citrus limon*) *EO* ΔΔ
Tea Tree (*Melaleuca alternifolia*)

- Use one or a combination of the above essential oils in the electric diffusor to disinfect the sick room air.

DIRECTIONS FOR INTERNAL USE

For a child at the onset of the disease:[39]
Eucalyptus *(Eucalyptus globulus)* EO
Hyssop *(Hyssopus officinalis)* EO ∆∆
Savory *(Satureja hortensis)* EO ∆∆

- Mix 6–8 drops of each of the above oils in a 2-ounce bottle vodka or brandy. Adjust dosage according to child's weight, using 5 drops of the essential oil/alcohol mixture for every 10 pounds of weight. Take with a half-glass warm water three times per day before meals.

For a child with the disease in full course:[40]
Cypress *(Cupressus sempervirens)* EO
Eucalyptus *(Eucalyptus globulus)* EO

- Add 10 drops of each of the above essential oils to a 2-ounce bottle of vodka or brandy. Adjust dosage according to the child's weight, using 5 drops of the essential oil/alcohol mixture for every 10 pounds of body weight. Add to a half-glass warm water. Also mix into the water the tinctures listed below:

Black currant *(Ribes nigrum)* HT
Burdock *(Arctium lappa)* HT ∆∆
Coltsfoot *(Tussilago farfara)* HT

- Adjust tincture dosage according to patient's age and weight. For children under the age of six, use 10 drops. For children between ages six and twelve, use 15–20 drops. For teens and adults, use 30 drops. Take combined mixture once every twelve hours.

Suggestions: *Give the patient bed rest and keep him warm. Avoid drafts. Drink fruit and vegetable juices rich in Vitamin C. To prevent or relieve earaches, see Ear Infections, p. 121. To disinfect the area around the eye, see Eye Infections, p. 125. For sore throats, see Sore Throat, p. 169. For fevers, see Fevers, p. 127.*

∆∆ Burdock HT: may enhance the effect of insulin or blood sugar lowering medications.

ΔΔ Hyssop EO: contraindicated for pregnancy and epilepsy.
ΔΔ Lemon EO: do not go into direct sunlight after applying on the skin.
ΔΔ Savory EO: contraindicated for pregnancy. Do not apply undiluted to the skin.

MOUTH INFECTIONS

The mouth is a sensitive area of the body where bacterial, fungal, or viral infections frequently occur. Although disease germs may invade the mouth, many other factors can result in symptoms. They include systemic diseases or diseases elsewhere in the body (e.g., measles, scarlet fever, syphilis), nutritional deficiencies, blood disorders, heavy metal poisoning, irritants such as alcohol, tobacco, hot foods and spices, and trauma or injury.

Gingivitis is inflammation of the gums, an early stage in the development of periodontal disease. It is characterized by redness, swelling, and the tendency to bleed. Gingivitis may be caused by poor dental hygiene, poorly fitting dentures or dental appliances, or can accompany upper respiratory infections.

Next to the common cold, periodontal disease is the second most prevalent infectious illness in the U.S. It affects up to 50 percent of the population over the age of 50. Periodontal disease is a disorder of the gums surrounding the teeth.

Plaque is caused by a gummy mass of microorganisms that adhere to the teeth. When left unchecked, the gums become infected and swollen and dental caries are likely. This leads to *pyorrhea*, an advanced stage of periodontal disease where the bone supporting the teeth begins to erode, the dental pulp becomes infected, and abscesses are likely.

Stomatitis is an inflammation of the tissues of the mouth. It affects the lips, the palate, and the inside lining of the cheeks with a diffuse, red swelling. The gums swell, bleeding easily.

Tiny ulcers called *canker sores* may form on the mucosa of the mouth. *Cold sores*, also called fever blisters may appear. Unlike canker sores, cold sores form blisters and are caused by the Herpes simplex virus.

Thrush is a stomatitis caused by a yeast fungus, *Candida albicans*. Characteristic symptoms include ulcers and milk-white patches on the tongue, mouth, and throat. It is usually accompanied by fever and gastrointestinal upset. It is common in infants and young children.

DIRECTIONS FOR INTERNAL USE
Fresh lemon juice

- To remove thrush from the mouth, rinse with a mixture of fresh lemon juice, honey, and water.[41]

Oral rinse:
Lemon *(Citrus limon)* EO

- To freshen the breath, rinse the mouth with a 2–3 drops how Lemon EO added to water. Also use Bergamot, Orange, Tea Tree or Thyme essential oil.

For temporary relief of gum and tooth pain:
Clove Bud *(Syzygium aromaticum)* EO

- Mix 1 part Clove Bud to 4 parts carrier oil. Using a cotton swab, apply the mixture directly on the area of pain.[42]
- As an alternative, add 1 drop Clove Bud to a toothbrush before adding toothpaste, then brush. Add 1 or 2 drops to your toothbrush in order to disinfect the toothbrush and to enhance oral hygiene

For mouth and gum infections:
Tea Tree *(Melaleuca alternifolia)* EO

- Add 2–4 drops Tea Tree essential oil to a glass of warm water. Mix well, and rinse the mouth and/or gargle two times per day, morning and evening.[43]

Disinfecting herbal mouthwash for gingivitis or periodontal disease:
Blackberry Leaf *(Rubus fruticosus)* HT ΔΔ
Calendula *(Calendula officinalis)* HT
Clove Bud *(Syzygium aromaticum)* EO
Lavender *(Lavandula augustifolia)* EO
Peppermint *(Mentha piperita)* EO ΔΔ

- To make a mouthwash, add 3–5 drops Lavender, 2–3 drops each of Clove Bud and Peppermint, 10–30 drops Blackberry Leaf, and 10–30 drops Calendula to a glass of water. Use 3 times per day.[44]

Suggestions: *Using commercial mouthwashes is not recommended. Most contain no more than alcohol, dye, and a flavoring. They irritate the gums and sensitive membranes of the mouth. They may temporarily kill the bacteria that cause bad breath, but they can also make the condition worse as bacteria return in greater virulence and strength than before.*[45]

ΔΔ Blackberry Leaf HT: if ingested, may cause nausea in some people.
ΔΔ Peppermint EO: contraindicated for pregnancy.

MUMPS

Mumps is a viral illness characterized by fever and inflammation of the salivary glands. It is primarily an acute childhood disease, occurring most often between the ages of 5 and 15. Mumps is spread by discharges from the nose and throat. It is less prevalent than measles and chickenpox, and less contagious.

Onset of the illness is gradual, and there may be chilliness, malaise, headache, pain below the ears, and moderate fever. Swelling affects the salivary glands in front of and below the ear. The lobe of the ear is sometimes pushed forward and the surrounding tissues fill with excessive body fluid. Facial features become distorted. Movements in the jaw are painful and restricted. These symptoms usually lasts from 5 to 7 days.

In adults, mumps can cause complications such as swelling in the testes, ovaries, and pancreas; inflammation of the brain and its meninges, and in rare cases, permanent impairment of hearing. Adults and teens should not needlessly expose themselves to the disease because serious complications may result.

INSTRUCTIONS FOR EXTERNAL APPLICATION
Ginger Root *(Zingiber officinale) EO*
Lavender *(Lavandula augustifolia) EO*

- Mix 3–5 drops Ginger Root or Lavender with a teaspoon of

carrier oil, massage over the salivary glands and bottoms of feet. Also effective if used with hot compress.

DIRECTIONS FOR INTERNAL USE

For mumps in a prepubescent child:
Ginger Root *(Zingiber officinale) EO*
Lavender *(Lavandula augustifolia) EO*

- Mix 15 drops of each of the above essential oils into a 2-ounce bottle of vodka or brandy. Adjust dosage according to the child's weight, using 5 drops of the essential oil/alcohol mixture for every 10 pounds of body weight. Add to a half-glass warm water. Also mix into the water the tinctures listed below:

Fumitory *(Fumaria officinalis) HT* ΔΔ
Blackberry Leaf *(Rubus fructicosus) HT* ΔΔ

- Adjust tincture dosage according to the patient's age and weight. For children under the age of six, use 10 drops. For children between ages six and twelve, use 15 to 20 drops. For older children and adults, use 30 drops. Take the combined mixture three times per day at mealtime.

For orchitis (inflammation of a testis) in a young adult:
Cypress *(Cupressus sempervirens) EO*
Eucalyptus *(Eucalyptus globulus) EO*
Savory *(Satureja hortensis) EO* ΔΔ
Thyme *(Thymus serpyllum) EO* ΔΔ

- Mix 11–12 drops Cypress, 11–12 drops Savory, 7–8 drops Eucalyptus and 7–8 drops Thyme into a 2-ounce bottle of Papaya tincture. Add 40 drops of this mixture into a half-glass of warm water. In addition, add 40 drops Elderberry *(Sambucus nigra)* tincture to the water. Take 3 times per day, before each meal.

Other useful herbal tinctures: *Calendula, Dandelion, Elderberry, Oat Straw, Red Clover.*

Other useful essential oils: *Eucalyptus, Geranium, Hyssop, Savory, Wild Rosemary.*

Suggestions: *Bed rest and a diet consisting of soft foods (warm cereal, vegetable puree, soup) because chewing and swallowing are often painful. Tart foods, such as pickles and lemon juice, may cause discomfort. Drink plenty of liquids including water, herbal teas, cranberry juice or currant juice.*

ΔΔ Blackberry Leaf HT: for people with weak stomachs, may cause nausea.

ΔΔ Fumitory HT: do not use in excess.

ΔΔ Savory EO: contraindicated for pregnancy.

ΔΔ Thyme EO: contraindicated for pregnancy, thyroid disorder, high blood pressure.

MUSCLE ACHES AND PAINS

Muscle aches and pain often accompany infectious illnesses. The pain may vary in intensity from mild discomfort to intolerable agony. A generalized aching over the entire body frequently accompanies influenza. Pain in the joints is a symptom of Lyme disease. A dull pain just below the last rib is often symptomatic of gallbladder infection.

INSTRUCTIONS FOR EXTERNAL APPLICATION

Black Pepper *(Piper nigrum)* EO ΔΔ
Clove Bud *(Syzygium aromaticum)* EO
Helichrysum *(Helichrysum angustifolium)* EO

• Mix essential oils with carrier oil, using a 10% dilution. Apply essential oil blend to area of pain or across the forehead and temples. If the pain does not subside within ten minutes, apply Helichrysum and Lavender neat.

Partial body massage for a child:
Lavender *(Lavandula augustifolia)* EO

• Massage the neck and shoulders using Lavender, apply neat.

To relieve joint pain:
Basil *(Ocimum basilicum) EO* ΔΔ
Carrot Seed *(Daucus carota) EO*
Fennel *(Foeniculum vulgare) EO* ΔΔ
German Chamomile *(Matricaria recutica) EO*
Roman Chamomile *(Chamaemelum nobile) EO*

- Mix one or several essential oils with a carrier oil, using a 10% dilution. Apply essential oil blend to area of pain. For instructions on preparing dilutions, see p. 82.

ΔΔ Basil EO: contraindicated for pregnancy.
ΔΔ Black Pepper EO: excessive use may overstimulate kidneys.
ΔΔ Fennel EO: contraindicated for pregnancy, young children, epilepsy.

PNEUMONIA

Pneumonia refers to an inflammation of the lung. In most cases, pneumonia results from a viral, bacterial, or fungal infection. Some types of pneumonia are not caused by infection, but by environmental factors such as exposure to chemicals and radiation. Other diseases may accompany pneumonia.

Viral pneumonia is most common among children and the elderly. Symptoms are similar to the symptoms of influenza. They include fever, dry cough, headache, muscle pain, weakness, high fever, and breathlessness.

Bacterial pneumonia is caused by the pneumococcus bacteria, a very serious illness. In severe cases, symptoms include shaking, chills, chattering teeth, severe chest pains, sweating, cough that produces rust-colored or greenish mucus, increased breathing and pulse rate, and a bluish tint to the lips or nails caused by a lack of oxygen. To fight the bacterial invasion, the lungs exudate (pour out fluids). The fluids fill the lung's air sacs, preventing the normal transfer of oxygen into the blood stream.

INSTRUCTIONS FOR EXTERNAL AND INTERNAL USE
See Bronchitis, p. 102.

Suggestions: *People with upper respiratory infections such as the common cold, middle ear infections, sinusitis, or bronchitis should seek prompt treatment for these conditions in order to prevent pneumonia from developing. Fatigue, chilling, over work and physical exhaustion, emotional stress, poor diet, and anything else that lowers the immune function should be avoided.*

PROSTATITIS

Prostatitis is an inflamed condition of the prostate gland. It may result from a long-standing bacterial infection, or as a complication of gonorrhea. Symptoms include a dull, aching pain in the perineal region, discharge from the penis, mild fever, pain, and difficult urination. Symptoms are more severe in the case of acute prostatitis. They include fever, chills, constipation, and vomiting, and frequent urination followed by the retention of urine. Medical consultation is required for all prostate problems.

Because of its tenacity, prostatitis should be treated with herbs and essential oils for an extended period of up to two months. Complementary treatments, including diet, exercise, and vitamin and mineral therapy are also important.

DIRECTIONS FOR INTERNAL USE
Ginger Root *(Zingiber officinale)* EO
Pine Needle *(Pinus sylvestris)* EO
Sandalwood *(Santalum album)* EO

- Mix 45 drops Ginger Root, 7 to 8 drops Pine Needle, and 7 to 8 drops Sandalwood into a 2-ounce bottle Papaya tincture. Add 40 drops of this mixture to a half-glass warm water, along with 13 drops of each of the following:

Lady's Mantle *(Alchemilla vulgaris)* HT
Uva ursi *(Arctostaphylos uva ursi)* HT

- Take the combined formula ten minutes before meals, three times per day.

Other useful herbal tinctures: *Bilberry, Buchu, Butcher's Broom, Couchgrass, Ginkgo, Goldenrod, Horsetail, Lady's Mantle, Saw Palmetto.*

Other useful essential oils: *Cypress, Lemon, Tea Tree, Thyme, Sage.*

Suggestions: *See Cystitis, p. 117, for dietary recommendations, add Vitamin B complex (50 mg 3 times daily) plus extra Vitamin B6 (50 mg 2 times daily). Drink teas made from diuretic herbs, such as Buchu, Juniper, Parsley, Slippery Elm, or Uva Ursi. Increase blood circulation through appropriate exercise or treatments such as hot baths and massage. Yoga is an excellent form of exercise for prostatitis.*

PSORIASIS

Psoriasis is a chronic skin rash characterized by discrete pink or dull-red lesions covered with scaling, patchy, silvery-looking skin. The plaques consist of large, raised lesions typically greater than 1 cm. in diameter. Psoriasis can affect just certain parts of the body, such as the knees, scalp, or elbows; or it can spread to many areas.

Psoriasis is not contagious. Symptoms can vary greatly in severity or frequency of occurrence.

What causes psoriasis is not known. Psoriasis often runs in families and usually develops gradually. Psoriasis can occur in conjunction with arthritis. A number of factors are thought to influence the progression of psoriasis, including the incomplete digestion of proteins, a toxic bowel, food sensitivities, poor liver function, reaction to alcoholic beverages, and eating high amounts of animal fats. Contributing factors include stress, sunburn, skin irritation, and skin creams.

Some researchers believe that psoriasis is caused largely by a fungal infection. The fungus itself is located in the skin lesions that are characteristic of psoriasis; however, it originates from within the body in the intestines. From there it is "seeded" to the skin. Endocrine disturbances, particularly adrenal disorders and hypothyroidism, may also play a role in causing psoriasis.

To resolve psoriasis, antifungal treatment must be directed at both the infected skin as well as the intestinal tract within the body.

INSTRUCTIONS FOR EXTERNAL AND INTERNAL USE

See Eczema, p. 123.

Suggestions: *Follow a low sugar or sugar-free diet, since fungus lives on sugar. Avoid all sugary foods, including starchy foods that convert to sugar in digestion (e.g., potatoes, grains, pasta). Instead, eat vegetables and foods rich in protein. Supplement the diet with essential fatty acids, vitamins, and minerals.*

SCARLET FEVER

Scarlet fever is a bacterial infection resulting in sore throat, strawberry tongue, fever, and a point-like rash on the body. The rash is seldom seen on the face. At times, scarlet fever may occur without any rash at all. The illness most commonly affects school children between the ages of 6 and 10. It attacks most frequently in the winter and spring. Scarlet fever is a serious condition if left untreated. Seek out medical care.

As a rule, the disease begins with a sore throat and elevated temperature from 101° to 105° F. (38.3° to 40.6° C.), and frequent vomiting. The rash follows within 12 to 36 hours, and appears first on the neck and chest. It then spreads over the rest of the body, including the extremities. The face is flushed and there may be a characteristic pallor around the mouth. The tongue is heavily coated and strawberry-red in color. The tonsils and parotid (salivary) glands are engorged and swollen. In most cases, these symptoms last two or three days before they subside.

Full recovery from scarlet fever lasts from three to six weeks. To avoid complications, insist on sufficient bed rest during the convalescent period. Continue using essential oils and herbs as indicated below for 5 to 6 weeks to ensure full recovery. Do not cut treatments short. [46]

DIRECTIONS FOR INTERNAL USE[47]

Clove Bud *(Syzygium aromaticum)* EO
Eucalyptus *(Eucalyptus globulus)* EO
Lavender *(Lavandula augustifolia)* EO
Savory *(Satureja hortensis)* EO △△

- Mix 4–5 drops of each of the above essential oils with a 2-ounce bottle vodka or brandy. Adjust dosage according to the child's weight, using 5 drops of the essential oil/alcohol mixture for every 10 pounds of body weight. Add to a half-glass warm water. Also mix into the water the tinctures listed below:

Borage *(Barrago officinalis) HT* ΔΔ
Couchgrass *(Triticum repens) HT*
White Ash *(Fraxinus excelsior) HT*

- Adjust tincture dosage according to the patient's age. For children under the age of six, use a total of 10 drops. For children between ages six and twelve, use a total of 15 to 20 drops. For older children and adults, use a total of 30 drops. Take the combined mixture two to four times per day.

Gargle to disinfect the mouth and throat:
Cinnamon Bark *(Cinnamomum zeylanicum) EO* ΔΔ
Lavender *(Lavandula augustifolia) EO*
Savory *(Satureja hortensis) EO* ΔΔ
Blackberry Leaf *(Rubus fruticosus) HT* ΔΔ
Calendula *(Calendula officinalis) HT*

- Add 20 drops each of Cinnamon Bark, Lavender, and Savory and 1 teaspoon each of Blackberry Leaf and Calendula tincture to a two-ounce bottle Sweet Almond oil. Add 10 to 20 drops of this mixture to a glass of warm water. Gargle, do not swallow, three times per day.

Air antiseptic:
Eucalyptus *(Eucalyptus globulus) EO*
Lavender *(Lavandula augustifolia) EO*
Lemon *(Citrus limon) EO*
Tea Tree *(Melaleuca alternifolia) EO*

- Use one or more of the above essential oils in an electric diffusor to disinfect the sick room air.

Other useful essential oils: *Black Pepper, Niaouli, Pine Needle, Thyme.*
Other useful herbal tinctures: *Black Currant, Gentian.*
Suggestions: *See Sore Throat, p. 169.*

ΔΔ Black Berry Leaf HT: ingestion may cause vomiting in people with weak stomachs.

ΔΔ Borage HT: check with doctor before using if you have a liver disorder.

ΔΔ Cinnamon Bark EO: contraindicated for pregnancy. Do not use undiluted on the skin.

ΔΔ Savory EO: contraindicated for pregnancy.

SHINGLES

Shingles or *Zona* is an acute infection caused by the varicella-zoster virus, the same virus that causes chickenpox.

A vesicular rash appears on the trunk, usually on one side of the body. The vesicles, known anciently as "the fires of St. Anthony" because of the pain they cause, spread as a narrow band along a sensory nerve.

Shingles tends to affect older people or people with a lowered immune response. Outbreaks near the eyes can cause blindness; seek medical attention.

The incubation period is from 7 to 21 days. The total duration of the disease from onset to complete recovery varies from 10 days to 5 weeks. If all the vesicles appear within 24 hours the total duration is usually short. In general, the disease lasts longer in adults than in children.

Nerve pain that persists after the rash has cleared is called *postherpetic neuralgia*.

If treatment is started early, herbal medicines can be very effective for shingles, with successful results in most cases within one or two weeks.[48]

INSTRUCTIONS FOR EXTERNAL APPLICATION

Bergamot *(Citrus bergamia)* EO ΔΔ
Eucalyptus *(Eucalyptus globulus)* EO
Geranium *(Pelargonium graveolens)* EO
German Chamomile *(Matricaria recutica)* EO
Lavender *(Lavandula augustifolia)* EO
Tea Tree *(Melaleuca alternifolia)* EO

- Make a cold compress with one or more of the above essential oils and apply directly to the vesicles. If area is small, spot treat with undiluted essential oils. For example, use one drop each of Tea Tree and Lavender essential oils. Do not apply essential oils to the eyes. For larger areas, mix 5 drops each of Eucalyptus, Bergamot, and Tea Tree into 25ml of alcohol and apply to the affected area.[49]

Roman Chamomile *(Chamaemelum nobile)* EO

• For postherpetic neuralgia, apply Roman Chamomile essential oil topically to the area of pain.[50]

DIRECTIONS FOR INTERNAL USE
Lavender *(Lavandula augustifolia)* EO
Savory *(Satureja hortensis)* EO ΔΔ
Thyme *(Thymus serpyllum)* EO ΔΔ
Wild Rosemary *(Rosmarinus officinalis)* EO ΔΔ

• Mix 8–9 drops of each of the above essential oils into a two-ounce bottle vodka or brandy. Take 25 drops of this mixture in a half-glass of warm water. Before swallowing, add 8–10 drops of each of the following tinctures:

Dandelion *(Taraxacum dens leonis or T. officinale)* HT ΔΔ
Nettle *(Urtica urens or U. dioica)* HT
Artichoke *(Cynara scolymus)* HT ΔΔ

• Take the combined mixture three times per day 10 minutes before each meal.

Suggestions: *Topical gels or ointments are also available commercially. Look for additive-free products. Do not use petroleum jelly or oil-based applications on vesicles as these may irritate the skin, seal in toxins, and prevent normal skin respiration. Eat a diet rich in foods containing B vitamins and vitamin C. Also see Chickenpox, p. 110; Herpes simplex, p. 137.*

ΔΔ Artichoke HT: Do not use if you are pregnant, have gallbladder disease, gallstones, liver disease, kidney disease, or if you're allergic to plants in the Asteraceae family.
ΔΔ Bergamot EO: do not go into direct sunlight after applying on the skin.

ΔΔ Dandelion HT: do not use without doctor's permission if you have ulcers or gastritis.

ΔΔ Savory EO: contraindicated for pregnancy, thyroid disorder, high blood pressure.

ΔΔ Thyme EO: contraindicated for pregnancy, thyroid disorder, high blood pressure.

ΔΔ Wild Rosemary EO: contraindicated for epilepsy and high blood pressure.

SINUSITIS

Sinusitis refers to inflammation of the paranasal sinuses. These are hollow spaces in the skull that drain into the nasal passages. They are lined with a mucous membrane that assists in the production of mucus for the respiratory tract. In addition, they lighten the skull bones and serve as a resonant chamber for the production of sound.

Sinusitis can come about as a result of viral or bacterial infection, allergies, structural abnormalities (such as a polyp, a cyst, or a deviated septum), a dental abscess, smoking, exposure to irritating fumes or smells, a weak immune system, or other predisposing factors.

Phytotherapy treatment for sinusitis aims to shrink the nasal mucosa to facilitate drainage and ventilation of the nasal cavities.

Sinusitis is a potentially dangerous condition that requires aggressive treatment and may require consultation with a health care professional.[51] It should be treated as soon as it appears. Sinuses that are clogged a long time invite infection. There is always a tendency for sinusitis to become a chronic condition.

INSTRUCTIONS FOR EXTERNAL APPLICATION

Eucalyptus *(Eucalyptus globulus)* EO
Lavender *(Lavandula augustifolia)* EO
Niaouli *(Melaleuca viridflora)* EO
Peppermint *(Mentha piperita)* EO ΔΔ
Pine Needle *(Pinus sylvestris)* EO
Thyme *(Thymus serpyllum)* EO ΔΔ
Wild Rosemary *(Rosmarinus officinalis)* EO ΔΔ

- Select one or several of the above essential oils. Put 8–10 drops essential oil on a handkerchief and inhale for 2 to 3 minutes frequently during the day. At night, put drops on the pillow.
- Dr. Valnet's formula for catarrh: Mix 100 drops Eucalyptus, 25 drops Lavender, 50 drops Pine Needle, and 50 drops Thyme into a 2-ounce bottle alcohol. Add between one teaspoon and one tablespoon of this mixture to a bowl of boiling water. Inhale 2 or 3 times daily for 8 to 15 days.[52]

DIRECTIONS FOR INTERNAL USE

For chronic sinusitis:[53]

Cinnamon Bark *(Cinnamomum zeylanicum)* EO ΔΔ
Eucalyptus *(Eucalyptus globulus)* EO
Pine Needle *(Pinus sylvestris)* EO

- Mix 30 drops Cinnamon Bark, 22 drops Eucalyptus and 15 drops Pine Needle into a 2-ounce bottle Papaya tincture. Add 40 drops of this mixture to a half-glass warm water. Also add 25 drops of each of the following tinctures:

Black currant *(Ribes nigrum)* HT
Elderberry *(Sambucus nigra)* HT

- Take this combined mixture three times per day before meals for up to 8 weeks.

Other useful essential oils: *Cajeput, Cedarwood Atlas, Lemon.*
Other useful herbal tinctures: *Angelica, Artichoke, Cayenne, Garlic, Goldenrod, Horsetail.*
Suggestions: *If using commercial nose drops and sprays for decongestion, limit their use or avoid them altogether. They can cause side effects including jitteriness, insomnia, and fatigue. They also become addictive and interfere with normal sinus functions.*[54] *Patients with acute sinusitis require 24–48 hours bed rest, a well-balanced diet, and liquids. Use the diffusor with Lemon, Eucalyptus, Lavender or another suitable essential oil in the sick room. The diet should include foods rich in minerals and vitamins, especially the B complex vitamins and Vitamin C. Drink lots of liquids. If you have a chronic condition, see dietary recommendations for Candida albicans. See p. 108.*

ΔΔ Cinnamon Bark EO: contraindicated for pregnancy. Do not use undiluted on the skin.

ΔΔ Peppermint EO: contraindicated for pregnancy. Do not apply undiluted to the skin.

ΔΔ Thyme EO: contraindicated for pregnancy, thyroid disorder, high blood pressure.

ΔΔ Wild Rosemary EO: contraindicated for epilepsy and high blood pressure.

SORE THROAT

A sore throat can be any inflammation of the tonsils, pharynx, or larynx. If one part of the throat is infected or inflamed, the other parts are almost certain to be affected as well.

Symptoms of a sore throat can be mild to severe. Early symptoms include a dry, scratchy feeling, a hoarse or husky voice, and excessive mucus discharge. Pain in the throat, headache, coughing, choking, difficulty talking or swallowing, and pain in the ears come next. The throat is red and swollen. Sometimes it has whitish-yellow spots.

In the case of an acute infection, a sore throat is usually accompanied by chills, fever, loss of appetite, and body aches and pains. Loss of voice is characteristic of laryngitis.

The infecting organism causing sore throat is frequently a streptococcus. However, there are many other organisms present in the upper respiratory tract. Sore throat or loss of voice can also be caused by an excessive use of the voice, smoking, or by exposure to dust, fumes, or other adverse environmental conditions.

Sore throats may signal oncoming colds, flu, mononucleosis, herpes simplex, or a childhood illness. In adults, sore throats may accompany diphtheria, rheumatic fever, polio, or cancer.

DIRECTIONS FOR INTERNAL USE

Cinnamon Bark *(Cinnamomum zeylanicum)* EO ΔΔ
Cypress *(Cupressus sempervirens)* EO
Eucalyptus *(Eucalyptus globulus)* EO
Lavender *(Lavandula augustifolia)* EO
Thyme *(Thymus serpyllum)* EO ΔΔ

For a sore throat, choose the treatment that best suits your needs:

- Take one drop of Cypress mixed with a teaspoon of raw honey every 15 minutes at first sign of sore throat. Do not use this oral method for children.[55]
- Add 3–5 drops Thyme to honey water, use 3 times per day. According to Valnet, this is "one of the best remedies."[56]
- Mix 18 drops Cinnamon Bark and 18 drops Lavender in a 2-ounce bottle vodka or brandy. Add 30 drops of this mixture to a half-glass of warm water and swallow. Use morning, midday, and at night.[57]

Suggestions: *See Common Cold, Fever, Influenza, Tonsillitis.*

ΔΔ Cinnamon Bark EO: contraindicated for pregnancy. Do not use undiluted on the skin.

ΔΔ Thyme EO: contraindicated for pregnancy, thyroid disorder, high blood pressure.

TESTICULAR INFECTION

Orchitis is an inflamed condition of the testicle. The inflammation may be a complication of venereal disease, tuberculosis, mumps, prostatitis, urethritis, surgery, or an infection elsewhere in the body. Symptoms include swelling, severe pain, fever and chills, vomiting, hiccough, and delirium.

The French doctors treat orchitis by rectal administration of essential oils and herbs. The plants listed here are for oral use. They are selected for their estrogen-like effects as well as their anti-inflammatory properties.

DIRECTIONS FOR INTERNAL USE

Cajeput *(Melaleuca cajeputi)* EO

Cypress *(Cupressus sempervirens)* EO

Fennel *(Foeniculum vulgare)* EO ΔΔ

Savory *(Satureja hortensis)* EO ΔΔ

Thyme *(Thymus serpyllum)* EO ΔΔ

- From the above list, select one or more essential oils. Mix 30 drops essential oils into a one-ounce bottle of herbal tincture, such as Calendula (*Calendula officinalis*), Hops (*Humulus lupulus*), or Elderberry (*Sambucus nigra*). For example, mix 10 drops each of Cypress, Fennel, and Savory to a 1 oz. bottle of Elderberry. Take 10 to 30 drops of this mixture, 3 times per day before meals.

Other useful herbal tinctures: *Angelica, St. John's Wort.*
Suggestions: *bed rest, support of scrotum (immobilize organ), use ice bag, suspend sexual intercourse.*

ΔΔ Fennel EO: contraindicated for pregnancy, young children, epilepsy.
ΔΔ Savory EO: contraindicated for pregnancy. Do not use undiluted on the skin.
ΔΔ Thyme EO: contraindicated for thyroid disorder, high blood pressure.

TONSILLITIS

The tonsils are small organs located on either side of the entrance to the throat. They act as a filter to protect the body from invasion. They also aid in the formation of white blood cells.

Tonsillitis, or inflammation of the tonsils, occurs as a result of bacterial or viral infection. Symptoms include sore throat, difficulty swallowing, hoarseness, coughing, redness, pain, and swelling. Onset is sudden, usually accompanied by chills, fever, malaise, headache, pains and aches in the back and extremities.

Tonsillitis is most common in children, but can occur at any age. Some people have repeated bouts as tonsillitis becomes a chronic condition. This can be difficult to cure, because each time as the tonsils become inflamed, scar tissue accumulates.

DIRECTIONS FOR INTERNAL USE
Blackberry Leaf (*Rubus fructicosus*) HT ΔΔ

* Add 10–20 drops Blackberry Leaf to a lukewarm glass of lemon water and gargle 3 or 4 times per day.

Cinnamon Bark (*Cinnamomum zeylanicum*) EO ΔΔ
Lavender (*Lavandula augustifolia*) EO

Savory *(Satureja hortensis)* EO ∆∆
Blackberry Leaf *(Rubus fructicosus)* HT ∆∆
Calendula *(Calendula officinalis)* HT

- Add 12 drops of each of the above essential oils and one teaspoon of each of the tinctures to a 2-ounce bottle of alcohol or Sweet Almond oil. Use as a gargle, 3 or 4 times per day or as often as needed.

Eucalyptus *(Eucalyptus globulus)* EO
Tea Tree *(Melaleuca alternifolia)* EO
Thyme *(Thymus serpyllum)* EO ∆∆

- Mix 12 drops of each of the above essential oils into a 2-ounce bottle Papaya tincture. Add 30 drops of this mixture into a half-glass warm lemon water. Also add 10 drops each of the following tinctures:

Agrimony *(Agrimonia eupatoria)* HT
Blackberry Leaf *(Rubus fructicosus)* HT ∆∆
Black Currant *(Ribes nigrum)* HT

- Take the combined mixture 3 times per day, before meals. If there is a lot a phlegm in the upper respiratory tract, use the following tinctures instead of those listed: Elecampane *(Inula helenium)* and Marshmallow root *(Althea officinalis)*.

Suggestions: *Give the patient bed rest for 24 to 48 hours, with lots of liquids to drink. The following juices are beneficial: Cranberry, Lemon, Celery, Cabbage. Include garlic, onions, figs and turnips in the diet. Supplement with Vitamin C and zinc lozenges. A recommended procedure is to take one 15 mg. zinc lozenge every 2–3 waking hours for the first 3 days, then reduce dosage to one lozenge 4 times per day until the condition clears.*[58]

∆∆ Blackberry Leaf HT: may cause nausea in people with weak stomachs.
∆∆ Cinnamon Bark EO: contraindicated for pregnancy. Do not use undiluted on the skin.

ΔΔ Savory EO: contraindicated for pregnancy.

ΔΔ Thyme EO: contraindicated for pregnancy, thyroid disorder, high blood pressure.

TUBERCULOSIS

Tuberculosis is a highly contagious disease transmitted through inhalation or swallowing droplets contaminated with the TB bacillus (*Mycobacterium tuberculosis*). It usually affects the lungs and surrounding tissues but can invade any other tissue or organ. Early stages of TB are characterized by fatigue, chest pain, weight loss, and fever. As the disease progresses, difficult or labored breathing may follow. Successful treatment of tuberculosis requires a combination of drugs for an extended period, usually longer than one year. Tuberculosis may develop as a chronic condition, lasting for years.

DIRECTIONS FOR INTERNAL USE

Peppermint (*Mentha piperita*) EO ΔΔ

Savory (*Satureja hortensis*) EO ΔΔ

Thyme (*Thymus serpyllum*) EO ΔΔ

- Mix 22 drops Savory, 8 drops Peppermint, 8 drops Thyme into a 2-ounce bottle vodka or brandy. Add 40 drops of this mixture into a half-glass warm water. Also add 10 drops of each of the following tinctures:

Black Walnut or English Walnut (*Juglans nigra or Juglans regia*) HT ΔΔ

Elecampane (*Inula helenium*) HT ΔΔ

White Oak (*Quercus alba*) HT

- Take the combined mixture three times per day before meals.

Phosphate of Soda (*Natrum Phosphoricum*)[59]

Phosphate of Magnesia (*Magnesia phosphorica*)

Phosphate of Lime (*Calcarea phosphorica*)

Fluroride of Lime (*Calcareafluorica*)

Silicic Acid (*Silicea*)

- Schussler cell salts are trace minerals needed by the body in minute amounts. The French doctors recommend these for tuberculosis. Take in addition to regular mineral supplementation.

Other useful essential oils: *Cedarwood Atlas, Clove Bud, Eucalyptus, Ginger Root, Hyssop, Pine Needle.*
Other useful herbal tinctures: *Garlic, Plantain.*
Suggestions: *Supplement with minerals, vitamins, enzymes, and essential fatty acids. Get plenty of rest and breathe fresh air. If possible, go to the country or mountains for a change of air. Drink at least one glass of freshly made vegetable juice per day. Cabbage, turnip, cress, and celery juices are especially important. Other raw, fresh vegetable and fruit juices are also good.*

ΔΔ Black Walnut HT: contraindicated for pregnancy.
ΔΔ Elecampane HT: contraindicated for pregnancy.
ΔΔ Peppermint EO: contraindicated for pregnancy.
ΔΔ Savory EO: contraindicated for pregnancy.
ΔΔ Thyme EO: contraindicated for pregnancy, thyroid disorder, high blood pressure.

URETHRITIS

Urethritis is an inflammation of the urethra often caused by an organism transmitted during sexual intercourse. Lab tests should be done to determine the infectious agent to be treated. The treatment varies accordingly.

DIRECTIONS FOR INTERNAL USE
For a common non-bacterial infection:[60]
Cajeput *(Melaleuca cajeputi) EO*
Fennel *(Foeniculum vulgare) EO* ΔΔ
Thyme *(Thymus serpyllum) EO* ΔΔ

- Mix 12 drops of each of the above essential oils into a 2-ounce bottle Papaya tincture. Add 40 drops of this mixture to a half-glass of water. Also add 13 drops of each of the following tinctures to the water:

Bilberry *(Vaccinium myrtillus) HT* ΔΔ

Bistort *(Polygonum bistorta)* HT △△
Goldenrod *(Solidago virgaurea)* HT

- Take the combined mixture before meals, three times per day.

For a bacterial infection:
See Vaginitis, p. 176.

For an infection caused by parasites (trichomonas):
Cajeput *(Melaleuca cajeputi)* EO
Tea Tree *(Melaleuca alternifolia)* EO
Thyme *(Thymus serpyllum)* EO △△

- Mix 22 drops Cajeput, 15 drops Tea Tree, and 30 Thyme into a 2-ounce bottle Papaya tincture. Add 50 drops of this mixture into a half-glass of Thyme tea. Also add 25 drops of each of the following tinctures into the tea:

Couchgrass *(Triticum repens)* HT
Uva Ursi *(Arctostaphylos uva ursi)* HT △△

- Take the combined mixture 5 times per day for the first two days, then 3 times per day for the next six weeks.

Note: to make Thyme tea, put freshly harvested Thyme leaves into a quart jar, cover with just-boiled water and let stand until it is cool enough to drink. If fresh leaves are not available, use the dried herb, ground or chopped. Strain the tea into cups.

For a yeast infection:
See Candida albicans, p. 108.
See Vaginitis, p. 176.

Other useful essential oils: *Cinnamon Bark, Oregano, Sandalwood.*
Other useful herbal tinctures: *Buchu, Elecampane.*
Suggestions: *See Cystitis, p. 117. Temporarily suspend sexual intercourse. Give sex partner the same treatment.*

Abbreviation Key: **HT**=HERBAL TINCTURE   **EO**=ESSENTIAL OIL   △△=CAUTIONS   **175**

ΔΔ Bilberry HT: diabetics check with doctor before using.

ΔΔ Bistort HT: can aggravate arthritis, rheumatism, gout in some people, use with caution.

ΔΔ Fennel EO: contraindicated for pregnancy, young children, epilepsy.

ΔΔ Thyme EO: contraindicated for pregnancy, thyroid disorder, high blood pressure.

ΔΔ Uva Ursi HT: contraindicated for pregnancy.

VAGINITIS

An infection resulting in inflammation of either the external female genitals and the vagina, or of the glands that secrete mucus on either side of the vaginal orifice. *Vaginitis* results from a change in the balance of vaginal bacteria. Symptoms include a milky discharge with a fishy odor. Vaginitis can lead to pelvic infection, infertility, or complications with pregnancy.

Thrush is a yeast infection of the vagina that results in itching, burning, and a white discharge resembling cottage cheese. Those most susceptible include people with food allergies, diminished immune response, and stress. The use of antibiotics and birth control pills has also been linked to this condition, since these upset the balance of intestinal flora which keep candida albicans under control.

A third type of vaginal infection is called *trichomoniasis*, a sexually transmitted disease caused by a parasite. Its symptoms include a fishy odor, heavy yellow-green or gray discharge, and painful intercourse.

As with other infections of the urinary tract and reproductive organs, the successful treatment of vaginitis requires first identifying the causative agent and adjusting the treatment protocol accordingly.

INSTRUCTIONS FOR EXTERNAL APPLICATION

Tea Tree *(Melaleuca alternifolia) EO*

- Mix 6–8 drops Tea Tree with a teaspoon of carrier oil. Apply to the lower abdomen or bottoms of feet, as often as needed.
- Apply 20 drops of mixture to the tip of a tampon. Insert for 4 hours, once a day for three days. Effective for vaginal yeast infections.
- Vaginal douche or enema: Add 10 drops Tea Tree essential oil to a quart of distilled water. Use to disinfect and to reduce discomfort and irritation.[61]

DIRECTIONS FOR INTERNAL USE

For a parasite infection (trichomonas):
Cinnamon Bark *(Cinnamomum zeylanicum)* *EO* ΔΔ
Ginger Root *(Zingiber officinale)* *EO*
Lavender *(Lavandula augustifolia)* *EO*

- Mix 24 drops of each above oil in a 2-ounce bottle Papaya tincture. Add 30 drops of this mixture to a half-glass of warm water. Also add 15 drops of each of the following tinctures:

Lady's Mantle *(Alchemilla vulgaris)* *HT*
Yarrow *(Achillea millefolium)* *HT*

- Take the combined mixture three times per day, before meals.

For a yeast infection:
Oregano *(Oreganum vulgare)* *EO* ΔΔ
Tea Tree *(Melaleuca alternifolia)* *EO*

- Select one or both essential oils. If using one essential oil, mix between 38 and 45 drops into a 2-ounce bottle vodka or brandy. If using two essential oils, mix 22 drops of each into the bottle. Add 30 drops of this mixture to a half-glass warm water. Also add 15 drops of each of the following tinctures to the water:

Buchu *(Barosma betulina)* *HT* ΔΔ
Goldenseal *(Hydrastis canadensis)* *HT* ΔΔ

- Take the combined mixture before meals, three times per day.

For a bacterial infection:
Lavender *(Lavandula augustifolia)* *EO*
Oregano *(Oreganum vulgare)* *EO* ΔΔ
Sandalwood *(Santalum album)* *EO*

- Mix 15 drops of each above oil in a 2-ounce bottle of vodka or brandy. Add 40 drops of this mixture into a half-glass warm water. Also add 20 drops of each of the following tinctures:

Bistort *(Polygonum bistorta) HT* ΔΔ
Horse chestnut *(Aesculus hippocastanum) HT*

- Take the combined mixture three times per day, before meals.

Suggestions: *See Cystitis, p. 117. Supplement the diet with probiotics (Acidophilus, Lactobacillus). Take them as directed by your health care practitioner. Hygiene is very important. Douche as recommended above. Temporarily suspend sexual intercourse.*

ΔΔ Bistort HT: can aggravate arthritis, rheumatism, gout in some people, use with caution.

ΔΔ Buchu HT: diuretic, should not be taken by pregnant women without doctor's permission.

ΔΔ Cinnamon Bark EO: avoid during pregnancy. Do not apply undiluted to the skin.

ΔΔ Goldenseal HT: do not use excessively (more than 3 times daily) or long term (longer than 7 days). Contraindicated for pregnancy.

ΔΔ Oregano EO: contraindicated for pregnancy. Do not apply undiluted to the skin.

WARTS

Warts are abnormal growths on the skin caused by infection of the human papilloma virus. Warts can appear anywhere on the body, but they usually appear on the hands, feet, and face. They are usually nonmalignant and if left untreated will often disappear. Warts indicate the immune system may be weak.

Warts can be transmitted from person to person by touching someone who has a wart or touching something they have touched. Warts can also be transmitted by going barefoot in public areas (such as a locker room) or by borrowing someone else's comb or hair brush. Some people are more susceptible to warts than others.

Common warts are thick and rough and are often seen on children's hands. Most often they occur on areas of the skin exposed to friction or trauma. They can also occur inside the larynx and cause hoarseness.

Flat warts are smooth, flat-topped bumps the color of skin. They are most often found on the hands or face or on the lower legs of women who shave.

Plantar warts are found on the bottom of the feet, resembling calluses with a hard, black center. They tend to be tender to the touch and often bleed. Plantar warts usually do not spread to other parts of the body.

Palmar warts are warts on the palm of the hand.

Genital warts (condyloma) can lead to serious health problems if they are left untreated. They are usually pink or red in color, and appear most often in clusters. They spread through sexual contact, or, in the case of infants, by being exposed to genital warts during birth. Genital warts have a long incubation period; it may take up to three months after contact before the warts appear.

See a doctor for genital warts, warts that are bleeding, painful, changing in shape or color, or if they are larger than a pencil eraser.

INSTRUCTIONS FOR EXTERNAL APPLICATION
Tea Tree *(Melaleuca alternifolia) EO*

- Apply topically, three times per day until results are seen. Be patient, this may take up to a month or six weeks.

DIRECTIONS FOR INTERNAL USE
Cat's Claw *(Uncaria tomatosa) HT* ∆∆
Echinacea *(Echinacea angustifolia or E. purpurea) HT* ∆∆
Pau d'Arco *(Tabebuia avellandedae) HT*

Other useful essential oils: *Cinnamon Bark, Lemon.*
Other useful herbal tinctures: *Elderberry, Garlic.*

∆∆ Cat's Claw HT: contraindicated for hemophiliacs, organ transplant patients, and pregnancy.
∆∆ Echinacea HT: do not take if you are allergic to ragweed.

WHOOPING COUGH
Whooping cough is an acute, infectious childhood disease caused by the bacillus *Bordetella pertussis*. The disease spreads by contact with other

infected children. The illness is sometimes confused with diphtheria. Whooping cough requires medical care.

The incubation period typically lasts from 7 to 10 days. The first symptoms resemble a common cold, with a slight fever, sneezing, a dry cough, irritability and loss of appetite. After about two weeks, a convulsive, violent cough appears that begins with several short coughs followed by a long, drawn-out breath and a characteristic whooping sound. The child's face turns bluish, eyes become congested, and veins become distended. Vomiting and hemorrhaging often accompany the paroxysmal cough. This lasts for several weeks, after which the coughing becomes less frequent and less violent. Full recovery may take several months.

INSTRUCTIONS FOR EXTERNAL APPLICATION
Lavender *(Lavandula augustifolia) EO*
Tea Tree *(Melaleuca alternifolia) EO*

- Depending on child's age, mix 1–5 drops essential oils with a teaspoon carrier oil, rub on chest and back or massage the full body.

For use in the diffusor to disinfect the house/room air:
Clove Bud *(Syzygium aromaticum) EO*
Lemon *(Citrus limon)* or Lime *(Citrus aurantifolia) EO* ΔΔ

- Add 20 drops Clove Bud to a 15 ml. bottle Lemon *(Citrus limon)* or Lime *(Citrus aurantifolia)* and use in an electric diffusor to disinfect the sick room air.

DIRECTIONS FOR INTERNAL USE[62]
Basil *(Ocimum basilicum) EO* ΔΔ
Cypress *(Cupressus sempervirens) EO*
Thyme *(Thymus serpyllum) EO* ΔΔ

- Mix 6 drops of each of the above essential oils into a two-ounce bottle vodka or brandy. Depending on child's age and weight, use between 10–30 drops of essential oil/alcohol mixture in a cup of warm water or juice, 3 times per day, before meals. Use 10 drops for a child under six years of age, 20 drops for a child between the ages of six and 12, and 30 drops for a child older than 12. Also add to the glass 10 to 15 drops of each of the following tinctures:

Grindelia *(Grindelia squarrosa)* HT
Sweet Violet *(Viola odorata)* HT

• Take the combined mixture 3 times per day.

Other useful essential oils: *Cedarwood Atlas, Frankincense, Hyssop, Niaouli, Peppermint.*
Other useful herbal tinctures: *Agrimony, Catnip, Horehound, Sundew.*
Suggestions: *See Bronchitis, p. 102. Drink lots of liquids, including herbal teas and fresh fruit and vegetable juices.*

ΔΔ Basil EO: contraindicated for pregnancy.
ΔΔ Lemon EO: do not go into direct sunlight after applying on the skin.
ΔΔ Thyme EO: contraindicated for pregnancy, thyroid disorder, high blood pressure.

WOUND HEALING

A wound is a break in the skin or in the continuity of the body's soft tissues, caused by violence or trauma. There are many different types of wounds. Minor cuts, scrapes, or abrasions are common, especially in children. There are also more serious wounds, such as lacerations, puncture wounds, and open wounds.

A contusion is a wound where the skin is not broken. The soft tissues underneath the skin are injured or bruised.

Depending on the type of wound and how it was caused, a wound may result in trauma with bleeding, pain, discoloration, inflammation, swelling, an increase in body temperature and loss of function. The wound may become infected, healing slowly or not at all.

Unless careful hygiene is applied, a wound or injury that becomes infected may develop gangrene, a condition where body tissues decay as a result of inadequate oxygen to the area. Symptoms include pain, swelling, and tenderness. As the infection progresses, the tissue changes color, usually from pink to deep red to gray-green or purple. A sickly odor emanates. Left untreated, gangrene can lead to death.

INSTRUCTIONS FOR EXTERNAL APPLICATION

For minor cuts and scrapes:
Lavender *(Lavandula augustifolia)* EO
Tea Tree *(Melaleuca alternifolia)* EO

- Apply Lavender or Tea Tree undiluted directly to the wound to disinfect, clean, and heal.
- For wounds, clean the wound with water, removing any foreign objects. Make a sterile dressing with 2–3 drops essential oils on a cotton pad. Apply pressure until bleeding stops. Then apply an adhesive bandage. The cotton pad soaked with essential oil should remain in contact with the skin. Do not allow the essential oil to be absorbed by the adhesive bandage. After two hours, change the bandage.

For contusions:
Helichrysum *(Helichrysum angustifolium)* EO

- Contusions require liberal applications of Helichrysum several times per day. Continue applications for days, if necessary, until the bruising clears. Helichrysum is especially effective for bruising, but Black Pepper, Geranium, or Hyssop may also be used.

Aloe Vera *(Aloe barbadensis)*
Calendula *(Calendula officinalis)*

- For minor wounds, apply Aloe or Calendula cream directly to the affected area, as often as needed.

Comfrey *(Symphytum officinale)* HT ΔΔ
Goldenseal *(Hydrastis canadensis)* HT ΔΔ

Gotu Kola *(Centella asiatica)* HT
Slippery Elm *(Ulmus rubra)* HT
St. John's Wort *(Hypericum perforatum)* HT

- For minor wounds, use any of the above tinctures in a cool compress.

DIRECTIONS FOR INTERNAL USE

Astragalus *(Astragalus membranaceus)* HT
Echinacea *(Echinacea angustifolia or E. purpurea)* HT ΔΔ
Garlic *(Allium sativa)* HT ΔΔ

- The above herbs help strengthen the immune response and benefit wound healing. Use according to label directions, or take 10–30 drops herbal tincture, three times per day with meals. For children, adjust dosages according to age and body weight. Use 10 drops for children under the age of six, 20 drops for children between the ages of six and twelve, and 30 drops for children older than twelve.

Other useful essential oils: Black Pepper, Geranium, German Chamomile, Hyssop, Lemon, Peppermint, Pine Needle.
Suggestions: *If pain or a fever resulting from a wound continues without relief, seek medical care. During period of wound healing, increase consumption of foods containing Vitamin E and Vitamin C. Vitamin E is found in dark green leafy vegetables, brown rice, eggs, oatmeal, soybeans, sweet potatoes, and wheat germ. Vitamin C is found in berries, citrus fruits, and green vegetables.*

ΔΔ Comfrey HT: do not take internally without doctor's permission.
ΔΔ Echinacea HT: do not take if allergic to ragweed.
ΔΔ Garlic HT: thins the blood, to not use without doctor's permission if you are taking anti-coagulant drugs.
ΔΔ Goldenseal HT: contraindicated for pregnancy, do not use excessively (more than 3 times daily) or long term (longer than 7 days).

Glossary

Adaptogen . . . . Balances and regulates body functions

Analgesic . . . . Deadens pain

Anthelmintic. . . . . . . Destroys parasitic intestinal worms

Antibacterial . . . . Destroys bacteria

Antifungal. . . . . Combats fungal infection

Anti-inflammatory . . Reduces inflammation

Antispasmodic . . . . . Prevents or relieves spasms

Antitussive . . . . Prevents or relieves coughing

Antiviral . . . . Inhibits growth of viruses

Astringent. . . . . Causes constriction of tissues

Carminative . . . . Relieves flatulence

Cholagogue . . . . Increases the flow of bile into the intestine

Decongestant . . . . . . Reduces congestion

Demulcent . . . . Soothes or softens the mucus membranes

Diaphoretic . . . . Increases perspiration

Diuretic . . . . Increases urine flow

Emitic. . . . . Induces vomiting

Emmenagogue . . . . . Promotes menstrual flow

Emollient . . . . Soothes or softens the skin where applied

Expectorant . . . . Loosens and clears mucus from the respiratory
system

Febrifuge. . . . . Regulates fever

GRAS . . . . Generally regarded as safe

Laxative . . . . Facilitates passage of bowel contents

Mucolytic. . . . . Breaks down mucus

Parasiticide . . . . Destroys parasites

Phototoxic . . . . In direct sunlight, causes skin irritation

Purgative . . . . Causes water discharge from intestines

Sedative . . . . Reduces activity, calms

Stimulant . . . . Temporarily increases functional activity

Styptic . . . . Stops bleeding, hemorrhaging

Tonic . . . . Strengthens and regulates body functions

Vermifuge. . . . . Expels intestinal worms

Vulnerary . . . . Helps wounds heal

Appendix A
Essential Oil List

Name	Medicinal Effects	Comments/Responsible Cautions
Basil (*Ocimum basilicum*)	anti-inflammatory, antiseptic, antiviral, slightly bactericidal, decongestant, hormone like	Safe oil provided the methyl chavicol content is low. Avoid during pregnancy.
Bergamot (*Citrus bergamia*)	antiseptic, antibacterial, antifungal, antiviral, antispasmodic, calming, stimulates secretions	Unless bergaptene has been removed, can irritate the skin when exposed to direct sunlight.
Black Pepper (*Piper nigrum*)	analgesic, antibacterial, antiseptic, antispasmodic, antiviral, carminative, decongestant, diuretic, expectorant, febrifuge	Use in moderation. May overstimulate kidneys.
Cajeput (*Melaleuca cajeputi*)	antispasmodic, antiseptic for the intestinal, pulmonary, and urinary system, anthelmintic, diaphoretic, carminative, expectorant, febrifuge, insecticide, sudorific, tonic	GRAS
Caraway Seed (*Carum carvi*)	antibacterial, antifungal, antiseptic, antispasmodic, carminative, digestive stimlant, diuretic, emmenagogue, expectorant, hormone like, mucolytic	May irritate skin. High ketone content, should not be ingested for a long period of time (more than two weeks, 3 times per day). Do not us if pregnant or nursing. Not for children.
Carrot Seed (*Daucus carota*)	antibacterial, antiseptic, anthelmintic, calming, decongestant, diuretic, emmenagogue	GRAS
Cedarwood Atlas (*Cedrus atlantica*)	antibacterial, antifungal, antiseptic, astringent, calming, decongestant, diuretic, mucolytic	Do not use if pregnant.
Cinnamon Bark (*Cinnamomum zeylanicum*)	antibacterial, antibiotic, antifungal, antiseptic, antispasmodic, astringent, antiviral, carminative, emmenagogue, raises body temperature	Avoid if allergic to cinnamon. Do not apply undiluted, irritates the skin and mucous membranes. Avoid during pregnancy.
Citronella (*Cymbopogon nardus*)	anti-bacterial, antifungal, antiseptic, anti-spasmodic, diuretic, febrifuge	May cause skin irritation. Do not use if pregnant.

What To Do When Antibiotics Don't Work

Name	Medicinal Effects	Comments/Responsible Cautions
Clary Sage (*Salvia sclarea*)	antifungal, anti-inflammatory, antispasmodic, calming, decongestant, lowers blood pressure, uterine tonic	Do not use if alcohol has been consumed. Avoid during pregnancy.
Clove Bud (*Syzygium aromaticum*)	antibacterial, antifungal, analgesic, antispasmodic, antiviral, air antiseptic, uterine tonic	May cause skin irritation. Raises blood pressure.
Cypress (*Cupressus sempervirens*)	antispasmodic, antibacterial, astringent, decongestant	Balancing, tonic for the sympathetic nervous system.
Eucalyptus (*Eucalyptus globulus*)	anti-inflammatory, antiseptic, antiviral, decongestant, expectorant, mucolytic	Stimulates sweating, reduces body temperature.
Fennel (*Foeniculum vulgare*)	antibacterial, analgesic, anti-inflammatory, antiseptic, diuretic, hormone like, increases sweating	Avoid using if you have epileptic seizures. Do not use if pregnant or with babies, and young children.
Frankincense (*Boswellia carteri*)	analgesic, antibacterial, anti-inflammatory, astringent, cell regenerator, expectorant, mucolytic	GRAS
Geranium (*Pelargonium graveolens*)	analgesic, anti-bacterial, antifungal, anti-inflammatory, antispasmodic, cell regenerator, decongestant, diuretic	Excellent balancer, eliminates waste and congestion. Strong antibacterial properties.
German Chamomile (*Matricaria recutica*)	analgesic, antibacterial, anti-inflammatory, antispasmodic, temperature-reducing	GRAS
Ginger Root (*Zingiber officinale*)	analgesic, antispasmodic, antiseptic, anti-inflammatory, calming, decongestant, hormone like, reduces temperature, vermifuge	GRAS
Grapefruit (*Citrus paradisi*)	antiviral, air antiseptic, calming, diuretic	Unlike other citrus oils, Grapefruit is not phototoxic.
Helichrysum (*Helichrysum angustifolium*)	antibacterial, antifungal, antiseptic, antiiflammatory, antitussive, astringent, cholagogue, diuretic, expectorant	GRAS
Hyssop (*Hyssopus officinalis*)	anti-inflammatory, antispasmodic, astringent, diuretic, expectorant, emmenagogue	Do not use if pregnant or have epilepsy.

Name	Medicinal Effects	Comments/Responsible Cautions
Juniper Berry (*Juniperus Communis*)	analgesic, antiseptic, antispasmodic, diuretic, regulates menstrual cycle, stimulates digestion	Do not use if pregnant or have kidney inflammation.
Lavender (*Lavandula augustifolia*)	analgesic, antibacterial, antifungal, anthelmintic, anti-inflammatory, antiseptic, antispasmodic, antiviral, decongestant	GRAS
Lemon (*Citrus limon*)	antibacterial, antiseptic, antifungal, antiviral, calming, diuretic, lowers blood pressure	Possibly phototoxic, do not go into direct sunlight after using on skin.
Lemongrass (*Cymbopogon citratus*)	antibacterial, anti-inflammatory, antifungal, antiseptic, diuretic	A possible skin irritant.
Lime (*Citrus aurantifolia*)	antiseptic, anti-inflammatory, antispasmodic, decongestant, mucolytic	Possibly photo toxic.
Marjoram (*Thymus mastichina*)	antibacterial, antiseptic, calming, decongestant, expectorant	GRAS
Myrrh (*Commiphora myrrha*)	antibacterial, antiviral, antifungal, astringent, immune system tonic, emmenagogue	Do not use if pregnant.
Niaouli (*Melaleuca viridflora*)	antibacterial, antiviral, analgesic, decongestant, immune system tonic	Strongly antiviral, Niaouli is excellent for all respiratory problems.
Nutmeg (*Myristica fragrans*)	antibacterial, antiparasitic, emmenagogue, uterine tonic	Do not use if pregnant. Can cause hallucinations.
Orange (*Citrus sinensis*)	antibacterial, antifungal, anti-inflammatory, carminative, decongestant	May be photo toxic. Do not go into direct sunlight after using on skin.
Oregano (*Oreganum vulgare*)	antibacterial, anti-fungal, antiviral, carminative, diuretic, expectorant, emmenagogue	Do not use if pregnant. Avoid long term internal use. Skin irritant.
Patchouli (*Pogostemon cablin*)	antibacterial, antifungal, antiviral, anti-inflammatory, carminative, diuretic, lowers fever	GRAS
Peppermint (*Mentha piperita*)	antibacterial, antiviral, analgesic, antispasmodic, tonic for digestion	Do not use if pregnant. Do not apply undiluted to the skin.
Pine Needle (*Pinus sylvestris*)	antibacterial, antifungal, anti-inflammatory, decongestant, diuretic, expectorant, cortisone like, hormone like	Possible skin irritant.

189

What To Do When Antibiotics Don't Work

Name	Medicinal Effects	Comments/Responsible Cautions
Roman Chamomile (*Chamaemelum nobile*)	antibacterial, anti-inflammatory, antiparasitic, antispasmodic, emmenagogue	GRAS
Rose Otto (*Rosa damascena*)	antiseptic, antispasmodic, antibacterial, calming, decongestant, diuretic, emmenagogue, hormone like	GRAS
Sage (*Salvia officinalis*)	antibacterial, antifungal, antiviral, antispasmodic, diuretic, emmenagogue, expectorant, mucolytic	Avoid if patient has a history of epileptic seizures. Do not use if pregnant or with children. Raises blood pressure.
Sandalwood (*Santalum album*)	antibacterial, anti-inflammatory, astringent, antiseptic, calming, diuretic, promotes vaginal secretions	GRAS
Savory (*Satureja hortensis*)	antibacterial, antiviral, astringent, antiparasitic, air antiseptic, expectorant, vulnerary	Do not use if pregnant. Dilute before using on skin.
Tea Tree (*Melaleuca alternifolia*)	antibacterial, antifungal, antiviral, anti-inflammatory, antiseptic, analgesic, decongestant, causes sweating	GRAS
Thyme (*Thymus serpyllum*)	antibacterial, antispasmodic, antiparasitic, diuretic, expectorant	Do not use if you have high blood pressure, thyroid disorder or are pregnant.
Wild Rosemary (*Rosmariunus officinalis*)	antibacterial, antifungal, antiviral, anti-inflammatory, analgesic, antispasmodic, decongestant, emmenagogue, expectorant, mucolytic	Do not use if you are an epileptic or have high blood pressure.

Appendix B
Herb List

Name	Medicinal Effects	Comments/Responsible Cautions
Agrimony (*Agrimonia eupatoria*)	astringent, blood purifier, cholagogue, diuretic, tonic and vulnerary	None known.
Aloe Vera (*Aloe barbadensis*)	emmenagogue, emollient, laxative, purgative, stimulant, tonic, vermifuge and vulnerary	Do not use orally for more than ten days. Do not use if pregnant, have hemorrhoids or irritable bowel syndrome.
Angelica (*Angelica archangelica*)	antispasmodic, carminative, diaphoretic, diuretic, expectorant, stimulant, tonic	Not recommended for pregnant women or persons with diabetes.
Artichoke (*Cynara scolymus*)	antirheumatic, cholagogue, diuretic	If you have gallbladder disease or gallstones, consult with doctor before using. Contraindicated for pregnant women, nursing mothers, people with liver or kidney disease, or persons with allergies to plants in the Asteraceae family.
Astragalus (*Astragalus membranaceus*)	febrifuge, diuretic, tonic	GRAS
Barberry (*Berberis vulgaris*)	antiseptic, astringent, cholagogue, purgative	Use with caution. It should not be used with Glyccyrriza species (Licorice Root) because this nullifies the effects of the berberine.
Bilberry (*Vaccinium myrtillus*)	astringent, diuretic, tonic and antiseptic	Diabetics check with doctor before using.
Birch Bark (*Betula pendula or B. alba*)	anti-inflammatory, antirheumatic, antiseptic, astringent, diuretic, laxative	May be toxic to liver with extensive use.
Bistort (*Polygonum bistorta*)	astringent, demulcent, diuretic, febrifuge, laxative and strongly styptic	Use with caution if you have rheumatism, arthritis, gout, kidney stones.
Black Currant (*Ribes nigrum*)	diaphoretic, diuretic, febrifuge	None known.
Black Walnut (*Juglans nigra*) or English Walnut (*Juglans regia*)	astringent, blood tonic, emetic, laxative, vermifuge	No known hazards. Do not use if pregnant or nursing.

What To Do When Antibiotics Don't Work

Name	Medicinal Effects	Comments/Responsible Cautions
Blessed Thistle (*Cnicus benedictus*)	astringent, cholagogue, diaphoretic, diuretic, emmenagogue, tonic	No known hazards. Do not use directly on skin, or by people allergic to plants from the daisy family. May cause nausea.
Black Cohosh (*Cimicifuga racemosa*)	antirheumatic, antispasmodic, astringent, diaphoretic, diuretic, emmenagogue, expectorant, sedative	Poisonous in large quantities.
Boneset (*Eupatorium perfoliatum*)	antispasmodic, cholagogue, diaphoretic, emetic, febrifuge, laxative, purgative	Use with caution. Large doses are laxative and emetic.
Borage (*Barrago officinalis*)	diaphoretic, emollient, expectorant, febrifuge	The plant, but not the oil obtained from the seeds, contains small amounts of pyrrolizidine alkaloids that can cause liver damage and liver cancer.
Buchu (*Barosma betulina*)	diuretic	Should not be taken by pregnant women.
Burdock (*Arctium lappa*)	antibacterial, antifungal, carminative	Avoid if you have diabetes, low blood sugar, or use insulin.
Calendula (*Calendula officinalis*)	antiseptic, antispasmodic, astringent, cholagogue, diaphoretic, emmenagogue, vulnerary	GRAS
Cascara Sagrada (*Rhamnusd purshiana*)	laxative, tonic	Do not use if pregnant.
Cat's Claw (*Uncaria tomatosa*)	immune stimulant, anti-inflammatory, antiviral	Should not be taken by hemophiliacs, patients who have undergone an organ transplant, or by women who are pregnant or nursing.
Catnip (*Nepeta cataria*)	strongly antispasmodic, antitussive, astringent, carminative, diaphoretic, sedative	None known.
Cayenne (*Capsicum annum*)	antirheumatic, antiseptic, diaphoretic, rubafacient	Causes uncomfortable burning in the gastrointestinal tract for some people. Avoid accidental contact with eyes.
Celandine (*Chelidonium majus*)	antispasmodic, caustic, cholagogue, diaphoretic, diuretic, narcotic, purgative	Toxic, use with care.
Cleavers (*Galium aparine*)	astringent, diaphoretic, diuretic, febrifuge, tonic and vulnerary	Sap of the plant can cause contact dermatitis in sensitive people.

Name	Medicinal Effects	Comments/Responsible Cautions
Coltsfoot *(Tussilago farfara)*	antitussive, astringent, demulcent, emollient, expectorant, stimulant and tonic	The plant contains traces of liver-affecting pyrrolizidine alkaloids and is potentially toxic in large doses.
Comfrey *(Symphytum officinale)*	comfrey is especially useful in the external treatment of cuts, broken bones, bruises, sprains, sores, eczema, varicose veins	For external use only. Toxic to the liver if taken internally.
Couchgrass *(Triticum repens)*	demulcent, diuretic, emollient and tonic	None known.
Cranberry *(Vaccimium macrocarpon)*	used as a preventive against urinary tract infections	None known. Do not use tincture if you are also taking drugs for urinary tract infections or for kidney problems.
Dandelion *(Taraxacum dens leonis or T. officinale)*	cholagogue, strongly diuretic, laxative, tonic, an antibiotic against yeast infections	Use only under medical supervision if you have stomach ulcers or gastritis
Echinacea *(Echinacea angustifolia or E. purpurea)*	adaptogen, antiseptic, diaphoretic	Echinacea is best used at onset of illness. Not for prolonged use. People allergic to ragweed should avoid this herb.
Elderberry *(Sambucus nigra)*	antiviral, induces sweating, relieves constipation	GRAS
Elecampane *(Inula helenium)*	anthelmintic, antiseptic, astringent, bitter, cholagogue, demulcent, diaphoretic, diuretic, mildly expectorant, tonic	None known. Do not use if pregnant.
Eye bright *(Euphrasia officinales)*	astringent, herb of choice in the treatment of eye infections, also useful for respiratory system	GRAS
Fumitory Root *(Fumaria officinalis)*	antispasmodic, cholagogue, slightly mildly diuretic, laxative	Caution should be used. Laxative, excessive doses cause hypnotic and sedative effects.
Garlic *(Allium sativum)*	anthelmintic, antiseptic, antispasmodic, cholagogue, diaphoretic, diuretic, expectorant, febrifuge, stimulant	If you use anticoagulant drugs, check with your doctor before using Garlic.
Gentian *(Gentiana lutea)*	anthelmintic, anti-inflammatory, antiseptic, bitter tonic, cholagogue, emmenagogue, febrifuge	Use with caution if you have high blood pressure or gastric or duodenal ulcers.

193

What To Do When Antibiotics Don't Work

Name	Medicinal Effects	Comments/Responsible Cautions
Goldenrod (*Solidago virgaurea*)	antifungal, anthelmintic, anti-inflammatory, antiseptic, astringent, carminative, diaphoretic, febrifuge	GRAS
Goldenseal (*Hydrastis canadensis*)	antiseptic, astringent, cholagogue, diuretic, laxative, tonic	Do not use with low blood sugar or hypertension, or if pregnant or nursing.
Gotu Kola (*Centella asiatica*)	anti-inflammatory, febrifuge, nerve tonic	Skin irritant.
Grindelia (*Grindelia robusta*)	antispasmodic blood purifier, demulcent, expectorant, sedative	GRAS
Hawthorne Berry (*Crataegus oxyacantha*)	heart tonic, alleviates hypertension, irregular heart beat, atherosclerosis	GRAS, avoid combining with pharmaceutical drugs.
Heartsease (*Viola Tricolor*)	anti-inflammatory, demulcent, diaphoretic, diuretic, emollient, expectorant, laxative and vulnery	GRAS
Hops (*Humulus lupulus*)	antiseptic, antispasmodic, diuretic, febrifuge, sedative	Skin and eye irritant.
Horehound (*Marrubium vulgare*)	antiseptic, antispasmodic, cholagogue, diaphoretic, digestive, diuretic, emmenagogue, strongly expectorant	Avoid using if you have a heart disease.
Horse chestnut (*Aesculus hippocastanum*)	anti-inflammatory, astringent, diuretic, febrifuge, narcotic, tonic	Poisonous plant, use only after poisons have been removed as in commercial preparations.
Horsetail (*Equisetum arvense*)	antiseptic, astringent, carminative, diaphoretic, diuretic, vulnery	Do not use if pregnant. Use for short periods of time.
Juniper (*Juniperus communis*)	antiseptic, purifies blood, diuretic	Do not use if you have kidney disease. Not for long-term use (more than 6 weeks). Do not use if pregnant.
Khella (*Ammi visnaga*)	antispasmodic, diuretic	Phototoxic, may cause dematitis in some people.
Lady's Mantle (*Alchemilla vulgaris*)	antirheumatic, astringent, diuretic, emmenagogue, febrifuge, sedative, tonic and vulnery	GRAS
Licorice root (*Glycyrrhiza glabra*)	anti-inflammatory, antispasmodic, antiviral, diuretic, emollient, expectorant, laxative	Avoid if you have hypertension, liver disease, diabetes, hypokalemia, edema or rapid heart beat, or if you are taking dioxin-based drugs.

194

Name	Medicinal Effects	Comments/Responsible Cautions
Linden (*Tilia europa*)	antispasmodic, cholagogue, diaphoretic, diuretic, emollient, expectorant, sedative	GRAS
Lobelia (*Lobelia inflata*)	antiasthmatic, antispasmodic, diaphoretic, diuretic, emetic, expectorant and nervine	Do not use daily or on a regular basis. Not for children, pregnant women, or nursing mothers
Lomatium (*Lomatium dissectum*)	antibacterial, antiviral, mucolytic	Avoid if you are taking blood thinning drugs. Do not take in large doses. May cause rash.
Madder Root (*Rubia tinctorum*)	astringent, cholagogue, diuretic and emmenagogue	Do not use if pregnant.
Marshmallow (*Althaea officinalis*)	antitussive, demulcent, diuretic, highly emollient, slightly laxative	GRAS
Milk Thistle (*Sylybum marianum*)	astringent, bitter, cholagogue, diaphoretic, diuretic, emetic, emmenagogue, tonic	Concentrates nitrates, may cause cancer if used in excess.
Mullein (*Verbascum thapsus*)	anti-inflammatory, antiseptic, antispasmodic, astringent, diuretic, emollient, expectorant and vulnerary	GRAS
Nettle (*Urtica urens or U. dioica*)	antiasthmatic, antidandruff, astringent, depurative, diuretic, stimulating tonic	GRAS
Oregon Grape (*Berberis aquifolium*)	blood tonic, cholagogue, diuretic, laxative	Do not use for prolonged periods of time, in large doses, or if pregnant or nursing.
Papaya (*Carica papaya*)	antifungal, antioxidant, used to promote the digestion of proteins	GRAS
Parsley (*Petroselinum crispum*)	natural vitamin and mineral supplement, restorative, stimulating tonic, reduces blood pressure	Parsley leaf tea is recommended for urinary tract infections. Parsley seeds and essential oils should not be ingested.
Pau d'Arco (*Tabebuia avellandedae* or *Tecoma impetiginosa*)	antibacterial, antifungal, antiviral	In rare cases, causes nausea and diarrhea. Generally regarded as safe.
Plantain (*Plantago major*)	astringent, diuretic, expectorant	GRAS
Pleurisy root (*Asclepias tuberosa*)	antispasmodic, carminative, diaphoretic, diuretic, expectorant, tonic	Do not use if pregnant or nursing.

195

What To Do When Antibiotics Don't Work

Name	Medicinal Effects	Comments/Responsible Cautions
Purple Loosestrife (*Lythrum salicaria*)	antibacterial, highly astringent, vulnerary	GRAS
Red Clover (*Trifolium pratense*)	antispasmodic, diuretic, expectorant, sedative and tonic	GRAS
Red Raspberry (*Rubus idaeus*)	anti-inflammatory, astringent, decongestant	Avoid using large amounts. May cause loose stools or mild nausea.
Schizandra (*Schisandra chinensis*)	antitussive, astringent, cholagogue, expectorant, sedative, tonic	Do not use if pregnant or nursing.
Slippery Elm (*Ulmus rubra*)	anti-inflammatory, diuretic, expectorant	GRAS
Sundew (*Drosera rotundifolia*)	antibacterial, antispasmodic, antitussive, expectorant	GRAS
Sweet Violet (*Viola odorata*)	anti-inflammatory, diaphoretic, diuretic, emollient, expectorant, and laxative	GRAS
Teasel (*Dipsacus sylvestris*)	diaphoretic, diuretic	GRAS
Uva ursi (*Arctostaphylos uva ursi*)	antiseptic, astringent, diuretic, tonic	Do not use if pregnant. May be toxic.
White Oak (*Quercus alba*)	antiseptic and astringent	None known.
White Willow (*Salix alba*)	anti-inflammatory, antiseptic, astringent, diaphoretic, diuretic, febrifuge, sedative and tonic	Do not use if pregnant or nursing or have ulcers, allergic to aspirin or diabetes.
Wild Cherry Bark (*Prunus Serotina*)	antitussive, astringent, sedative	Do not use excessively.
Wormwood (*Artemisia absinthium*)	anthelmintic, anti-inflammatory, antiseptic, antispasmodic, carminative, cholagogue, emmenagogue, febrifuge, tonic, vermifuge	Do not use if pregnant or nursing. May cause nervousness, convulsions, insomnia, headaches. Toxic. Use with caution.
Yarrow (*Achillea millefolium*)	antiseptic, antispasmodic, astringent, carminative, cholagogue, diaphoretic, emmenagogue, vulnerary	May be photo toxic and cause skin irritation.
Yellow dock (*Rumex crispus*)	astringent, cholagogue	May cause mild diarrhea or nausea. Do not use if pregnant or nursing.

Notes

Endnotes—Introduction

Opening quotation from Shirley Price and Les Price, <u>Aromatherapy For Health Professionals</u>, Churchill Livingstone, 2nd. Edition, 1999.

1. Julia Lawless, <u>The Complete Illustrated Guide to Aromatherapy</u>, Element Books, 1997, p. 88.

Endnotes—Chapter 1

Opening quotation from Cecilia Salvesen, <u>Aromatherapy For Natural Health and Beauty</u>, Natural Health and Beauty College, Pinetown, South Africa, 2000.

1. Mathew Wood, The Book of Herbal Wisdom, Using Plants As Medicines, North Atlantic Books, Berkeley, California, 1997, pp. 12–13.
2. Ibid.
3. Ibid., pp. 219–220, 460.
4. Ibid. p., 244.
5. Ibid., p. 245.
6. Michael Castleman, <u>The New Healing Herbs</u>, Rodale, Inc., 2001, p. 168.
7. Shirley Price and Les Price, <u>Aromatherapy For Health Professionals</u>, Churchill Livingstone, 2nd. Edition, 1999., p. 9.
8. Cecilia Salvesen, <u>Aromatherapy For Natural Health and Beauty</u>, Natural Health and Beauty College, Pinetown, South Africa, 2000, p. 27.
9. Shirley Price and Les Price, op. cit., p. 26.
10. Kurt Schnaubelt, <u>Aromatherapy Course</u>, 3rd. Ed., Pacific Institute, 1985., p. II–18.
11. Kurt Schnaubelt, <u>Medical Aromatherapy, Healing with Essential Oils</u>, Frog Ltd., North Atlantic Books, p. 163.
12. Kurt Schnaubelt, <u>Advanced Aromatherapy, The Science of Essential Oil Therapy</u>, Healing Arts Press, Rochester, Vermont, 1998., p. 27.
13. Shirley Price and Les Price, op. cit., p. 25.

14. AV Rao and S. Agarwal, "Nutrition Research 19: (2) 305–323. February 1999.
15. Castleman, op. cit., p. 36.

Endnotes—Chapter 2
Opening quotation is from Barbara Hey, "The Illustrated Book of Herbs," Crescent Books, 1996.

1. Julia Lawless, The Complete Illustrated Guide to Aromatherapy, Element Books, 1997, p. 89.
2. Valnet, Jean M.D., Robert Tisserand (ed.) The Practice of Aromatherapy, A classic Compendium of Plant Medicines & Their Healing Properties, Healing Arts Press, Rochester, Vermont, 1980, p. 34.
3. Ibid., pp. 34 – 42.
4. Ibid.
5. Ibid.
6. Christian Duraffourd, Jean–Claude Lapraz, Jean Valnet, ABC de la Phytotherapie dans les maladies infectieuses, Jacques Grancher, (ed.), 1998.
7. Paul Belaiche, "Traite de Phytotherapie et d'aromatherapie Tome I— L'aromatogramme." Maloine S.A., Paris (1979)
8. C. Duraffourd, J.C. Lapraz, R. Chemli, La plante medicinale de la tradition a la science, 1er Congres Intercontinental, Plantes Medicinales et Phytotherapie, Jacques Grancher, Paris, 1997.
9. Ibid., pp. 170–184.
10. Cass Ingram, D.O., The cure is in the cupboard, how to use oregano for better health. Knowledge House, 1997., p. 6.
11. Kurt Schnaubelt, Advanced Aromatherapy, The Science of Essential Oil Therapy, Healing Arts Press, Rochester, Vermont, 1998, p. 83.
12. C. Duraffourd, J.C. Lapraz, R. Chemli, op. cit., pp. 170–184.
13. Annette Davis, telephone conversation, 04/01/02.
14. Julia Lawless, The Illustrated Encyclopedia of Essential Oils, Element Books, 1995, p. 228.
15. Cecilia Salvesen, Aromatherapy For Natural Health and Beauty, Natural Health and Beauty College, Pinetown, South Africa, 2000, p. 62.

16. Julia Lawless, <u>Tea Tree Oil, Nature's Miracle Healer</u>, Thorsons, 2001.
17. Reuters Health, February 15, 2002.
18. Rita Elkins, <u>The Pocket Herbal Reference</u>, Woodland Publishing, 2002.
19. Michael Castleman, <u>The New Healing Herbs</u>, Rodale, Inc., 2001, p. 196.
20. Ibid., p. 225.
21. Ibid., p. 227
22. Rita Elkins, op. cit., p. 91.
23. Ibid., p. 129.
24. Castleman, op. cit., p. 156.
25. Elkins, op. cit., p. 74.
26. Susan J. Murch, Sankaran KrishnaRaj, and Praveen K. Saxena, "Phytopharmaceuticals: Problems, Limitations, and Solutions." Scientific Review of Alt Med 4 (2):33–37,2000. Prometheus Books.
27. Ibid.
28. Marcia Angell and Jerome P. Kassirer, "Alternative Medicine: The Risk of Untested and Unregulated Remedies," <u>The New England Journal of Medicine</u>, 339, No. 12 (September 17, 1998):839–41.
29. Kurt Schnaubelt, Aromatherapy Course, 3rd. Ed., Pacific Institute, 1985., p. III–10.

Endnotes—Chapter 3

Opening quotation is from Mathew Wood, The Book of Herbal Wisdom, Using Plants As Medicines, North Atlantic Books, Berkeley, California, 1997.

1. National Intelligence Council, "The Global Infectious Disease Threat and Its Implications for the United States.", <u>www.cia.gov/cia/publications/nie/report/nie99-17d.html. p. 2</u>
2. Ibid.
3. <u>National Geographic</u>, "War on Disease," February 2002, p. 11.
4. National Intelligence Council, op. cit., p. 1
5. Ibid., p. 3
6. Ibid., pp. 1–37.
7. Ibid., p. 4
8. Ibid., p. 5

9. Ibid., p. 3

10. August 8, 2000. Bob Arnaut's Healthwatch on msnbc.com.

11. National Intelligence Council, op. cit., p. 3.

12. Gannett News Service, "Results of Attack Simulatons Aren't Encouraging," Salt Lake Tribune, March 10, 2002.

13. Mike Madden, Gannett News Service, "Hospitals Unprepared for Bioterror," Salt Lake Tribune, March 10, 2002.

14. Jeffrey Kluger, "A Public Mess," Time Magazine, January 21, 2002, p. 92.

15. National Intelligence Council, op. cit., p. 27

16. Michael D. Lemonick and Alice Park, "Vaccines Stage A Comeback," Time Magazine, January 21, 2002, p.70.

17. National Intelligence Council, op. cit., p. 23.

18. Leon Chaitow, Antibiotic Crisis, Antibiotic Alternatives, Thorsons, 1998.

19. Ibid.

20. Marc Lappe, Ph.D., <u>When Antibiotics Fail</u>, quoted in Chaitow, op. cit.

21. Christine Gorman, "Playing Chicken With Our Antibiotics," Time Magazine, January 21, 2002, p. 98.

22. Elizabeth Lipski, <u>Digestive Wellness</u>, 2nd ed., Los Angeles, Keats Publishing, 2000.

23. Schnaubelt, op. cit., p. 4

24. Ibid.

25. Chaitow, op. cit.

26. Julia Lawless, <u>The Complete Illustrated Guide to Aromatherapy</u>, Element Books, 1997, p. 89.

27. The Centers for Disease Control and Prevention, "MRSA - Methicillin Resistant Staphylococcus aureus," <u>www.cdc.gov/ncidod/hip/aresist/mrsafaq.htm</u>.

28. Leon Chaitow, <u>Antibiotic Crisis, Antibiotic Alternatives</u>, Thorsons, 1998.

29. National Intelligence Council, "The Global Infectious Disease Threat and Its Implications for the United States.", <u>www.cia.gov/cia/publications/nie/report/nie99-17d.html</u>

30. The Centers for Disease Control and Prevention, "Drug-resistant Streptococcus pneumoniae Disease," <u>www.cdc.gov/ncidod/dbmd/diseaseinfo/drugresstreppneum_t.htm</u>.

31. Essential Science Publishing, Essential Oils Desk Reference, May 2000, p. 371.
32. Michael A. Weiner, Maximum Immunity, Houghton Mifflin, 1986.
33. Kurt Schnaubelt, <u>Aromatherapy Course</u>, 3rd. Ed., Pacific Institute, 1985., p. III–25.

Endnotes—Chapter 4

Opening quotation from Kurt Schnaubelt, <u>Medical Aromatherapy, Healing with Essential Oils</u>, Berkeley, California: Frog, Ltd., 1999.

1. Laurel Vukovic, <u>14-Day Herbal Cleansing, A Step-by-Step Guide To All Natural Inner Cleansing Techniques For Increased Energy, Vitality And Beauty</u>. Prentice Hall, New Jersey, 1998, p. 103.
2. Sierra Magazine, 1999.
3. Samuel Epstein, M.D., author of <u>The Safe Shopper's Bible</u> and <u>The Politics of Cancer Revisted</u>.

Endnotes—Chapter 5

Opening quotation is from Mathew Wood, <u>The Book of Herbal Wisdom, Using Plants As Medicine</u>s, North Atlantic Books, Berkeley, California, 1997.

1. Kurt Schnaubelt, <u>Advanced Aromatherapy, The Science of Essential Oil Therapy</u>, Healing Arts Press, Rochester, Vermont, 1998., p. 37.
2. Ibid., p. 96.
3. Shirley Price and Les Price,<u> Aromatherapy For Health Professionals</u>, Churchill Livingstone, 2nd. Edition, 1999, p. 92.
4. James F. Balch, M.D. and Phyllis A. Balch, <u>Prescription for Nutritional Healing</u>, 2nd edition, Avery Publishing, 1997.

Endnotes—Chapter 6

1. Julia Lawless, <u>Tea Tree Oil, Nature's Miracle Healer</u>, Thorsons, 2001, p. 39.
2. Ibid., p. 28
3. Ibid., p. 39.
4. Christian Duraffourd, Jean–Claude Lapraz, Jean Valnet, <u>ABC de la Phytotherapie dans les maladies infectieuses</u>, Jacques Grancher, (ed.),

1998, p. 315.
5. Ibid., p. 313.
6. Cecilia Salvesen, personal communication.
7. Cecilia Salvesen, <u>Aromatherapy For Natural Health and Beauty</u>, Natural Health and Beauty College, Pinetown, South Africa, 2000, p. 120.
8. Ibid.
9. Christian Duraffourd et. al., op. cit., p. 167.
10. Julia Lawless, op. cit., p. 54.
11. Cecilia Salvesen, op. cit., p. 238.
12. Christian Duraffourd et. al., op. cit., p. 167.
13. Joseph Pizzorno, N.D., <u>Total Wellness</u>, Prima Publishing, 1996, pp. 30–31.
14. Jean Valnet, Robert Tisserand (ed.) <u>The Practice of Aromatherapy, A classic Conpendium of Plant Medicines & Their Healing Properties</u>, Healing Arts Press, Rochester, Vermont, 1980, p. 153.
15. Cass Ingram, D.O., <u>The cure is in the cupboard, how to use oregano for better health</u>. Knowledge House, 1997, pp. 63–64.
16. Cecilia Salvesen, op.cit., p. 178.
17. James F. Balch, M.D. and Phyllis A. Balch, <u>Prescription for Nutritional Healing</u>, 2nd edition, Avery Publishing, 1997, p. 272.
18. Schuyler W. Lininger, Jr. (editor), <u>The Natural Pharmacy</u>, 2nd ed., Healthnotes, Inc., 1999, p. 70.
19. Christian Duraffourd et. al., op. cit., p. 206.
20. James F. Balch and Phyllis A. Balch, op. cit., p. 286.
21. Elizabeth Lipski, <u>Digestive Wellness</u>, 2nd ed., Los Angeles, Keats Publishing, 2000, p. 215.
22. Christian Duraffourd et. al., op. cit. p. 204.
23. Ibid. p.228.
24. Ibid., p. 272.
25. Ibid., p. 273.
26. Ibid., p. 272.
27. L. Hervieux M.D., "Aromatherapy for HIV-Positive Patients," published in proceedings from the First International Symposium on Integrated Aromatic Medicine, Grasse, France, 1998.
28. Christian Duraffourd et. al., op. cit., p. 267.
29. Ibid., p. 268.

30. Ibid., p. 224.
31. Ibid.
32. Ibid., p. 174.
33. Julia Lawless, op. cit., p. 73.
34. Cass Ingram, op. cit., p. 71.
35. James F. Balch and Phyllis A. Balch, op. cit., p. 371.
36. Cass Ingram, op. cit. p. 97.
37. James F. Balch and Phyllis A. Balch, op. cit., p. 373.
38. Mathew Wood, <u>The Book of Herbal Wisdom, Using Plants As Medicines</u>, North Atlantic Books, Berkeley, California, 1997, p. 238.
39. Christian Duraffourd et. al., op. cit., p. 254.
40. Ibid., p. 255.
41. Jean Valnet, op. cit., p. 153.
42. James F. Balch and Phyllis A. Balch, op. cit., p. 426.
43. Julia Lawless, op. cit., pp. 74–75.
44. Schuyler W. Lininger, Jr. (editor), <u>The Natural Pharmacy</u>, 2nd ed., Healthnotes, Inc., 1999, p. 74.
45. James F. Balch and Phyllis A. Balch, op. cit., p. 296.
46. Christian Duraffourd et. al., op. cit. p. 257.
47. Ibid.
48. Ibid., p. 277.
49. Cecilia Salvesen, op. cit., p. 126.
50. Kurt Schnaubelt, <u>Medical Aromatherapy, Healing with Essential Oils</u>, Berkeley, California: Frog, Ltd., 1999., p. 247.
51. James F. Balch and Phyllis A. Balch, op. cit., p. 476.
52. Jean Valnet, op. cit., p. 143.
53. Christian Duraffourd et. al., op. cit., p. 306.
54. James F. Balch and Phyllis A. Balch, op. cit., p. 478.
55. Kurt Schnaubelt, op. cit., p. 234.
56. Jean Valnet, op. cit., p. 195.
57. Christian Duraffourd et. al., op. cit., p. 283.
58. James F. Balch and Phyllis A. Balch, op. cit., p. 506.
59. Christian Duraffourd et. al., op. cit., p. 333.
60. Ibid., pp. 185–188.
61. Julia Lawless, op. cit., p. 90.
62. Christian Duraffourd et. al., op. cit., pp. 241–243.

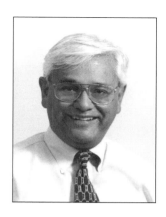

About the Author

Dirk van Gils is an author, teacher, and instructional designer. He was born in The Netherlands and has lived in Brazil, Indonesia, and Spain. He currently resides in the United States with his wife Toni. After receiving his Master of Science degree from Brigham Young University, he taught college and supervised the development of international training programs. Dirk speaks several foreign languages fluently.

In 1995, Dirk became the international sales manager for a company specializing in complementary and alternative medicine. He worked closely with alternative health care professionals from many countries, including naturopaths, herbalists, complementary health care physicians, nurses, and homeopaths. During this time he became interested in the medicinal use of aromatherapy and essential oils. Today, he devotes his time to writing, teaching, and research.